Roots of Wellness: Exploring Chinese Herbal Medicine

Traditional Wisdom for Modern Living

Olivia Bennett

© Copyright 2024 - All rights reserved.

The content contained within this book may not be reproduced, duplicated or transmitted without direct written permission from the author or the publisher.

Under no circumstances will any blame or legal responsibility be held against the publisher, or author, for any damages, reparation, or monetary loss due to the information contained within this book, either directly or indirectly.

Legal Notice:

This book is copyright protected. It is only for personal use. You cannot amend, distribute, sell, use, quote or paraphrase any part, or the content within this book, without the consent of the author or publisher.

Disclaimer Notice:

Please note the information contained within this document is for educational and entertainment purposes only. All effort has been executed to present accurate, up to date, reliable, complete information. No warranties of any kind are declared or implied. Readers acknowledge that the author is not engaging in the rendering of legal, financial, medical or professional advice. The content within this book has been derived from various sources. Please consult a licensed professional before attempting any techniques outlined in this book.

By reading this document, the reader agrees that under no circumstances is the author responsible for any losses, direct or indirect, that are incurred as a result of the use of information contained within this document, including, but not limited to, errors, omissions, or inaccuracies.

Table of Contents

INTRODUCTION 6

CHAPTER I: Fundamentals of Chinese Medicine 8

Yin and Yang: Balancing opposing forces 8

The Five Elements theory 10

Qi and Blood: Essential life energies in Chinese medicine

.... 13

CHAPTER II: The Role of Chinese Herbs 16

Understanding the principles of herbal medicine 16

Classifications of Chinese herbs 19

Methods of preparation and administration 21

CHAPTER III: Common Chinese Herbs and Their Properties

.... 25

Exploring popular herbs in Chinese medicine 25

Properties and therapeutic uses of each herb 28

How to incorporate these herbs into daily life 31

CHAPTER IV: Herbal Formulas and Prescriptions 34

Combinations of herbs for specific health conditions 34

Creating balanced and tailored herbal formulas 37

The holistic approach to addressing root causes 40

CHAPTER V: Diagnostic Methods in Chinese Medicine ... 43

Traditional diagnostic techniques (tongue diagnosis, pulse reading, etc.) 43

Understanding the body's signs and symptoms 46

Customizing herbal treatments based on individual assessments 49

CHAPTER VI: Chinese Herbal Medicine in Practice 53

Integrating Chinese herbs into a holistic wellness routine 53

Collaboration with Chinese medicine practitioners 56

Case studies illustrating successful herbal treatments 60

CHAPTER VII: Herbal Medicine for Modern Ailments 63

Addressing common health issues with Chinese herbs.... 63

Stress, insomnia, digestive problems, and more 66

The adaptogenic nature of many Chinese herbs 71

CHAPTER VIII: The Art of Herbal Healing 75

The connection between mind, body, and herbs.............. 75

Cultivating a mindful approach to herbal medicine 78

Herbal rituals and practices for overall well-being 82

CHAPTER IX: Sustainability and Ethical Considerations.. 86

Responsible sourcing of Chinese herbs 86

Environmental impact and conservation efforts 89

Ethical considerations in herbal medicine production .. 93

CHAPTER X: Challenges and Misconceptions 97

Addressing common misconceptions about Chinese herbal medicine 97

Overcoming skepticism and cultural barriers 101

Navigating challenges in integrating traditional practices with modern healthcare 105

CHAPTER XI: Future Perspectives and Innovations 110

Evolving trends in Chinese Herbal Medicine 110

Integration with modern medicine and scientific research 115

The potential for continued growth and development
.... 119

CHAPTER XII: Cultural and Spiritual Dimensions of Chinese Herbal Medicine 125

Chinese Medicine as a Lifestyle 125

Rituals and Practices for Holistic Living 127

Connecting with Nature and the Seasons 130

Exploring the Spiritual Essence of Herbal Medicine 132

CONCLUSION 136

INTRODUCTION

In a fast-paced world where wellness has become synonymous with modernity, "Roots of Wellness" invites readers on a profound journey into the time-honoured traditions of Chinese Herbal Medicine. This captivating book bridges ancient wisdom and contemporary living, unravelling the intricate tapestry of herbal remedies deeply rooted in Chinese culture.

As we navigate the complexities of modern health, "Roots of Wellness" emerges as a beacon, drawing on the profound knowledge embedded in Chinese Herbal Medicine. This book transcends the boundaries of a typical guide, inviting readers to explore the rich history, philosophy, and practical applications of herbal remedies that have endured for centuries.

The introduction unfolds like the delicate petals of a blossoming flower, revealing the essence of Chinese Herbal Medicine and its relevance to the challenges of our time. It beckons both novices and seasoned enthusiasts to embark on a journey where the wisdom of ancient herbal practices converges with the demands of contemporary living.

"Roots of Wellness" introduces the reader to the holistic principles that underpin Chinese Herbal Medicine, emphasizing the interconnectedness of mind, body, and spirit. The narrative weaves through the historical tapestry of herbal traditions, offering a deep dive into the cultural significance of various herbs and their applications in promoting wellness.

As the pages turn, readers are guided through the symbiotic relationship between nature and human health, unveiling the profound insights that have sustained Chinese Herbal Medicine through the ages. "Roots of

Wellness" is not merely a guidebook; it explores a holistic lifestyle, where traditional wisdom becomes a compass for navigating the complexities of modern well-being. Join us on this immersive journey, where ancient roots intertwine with the pursuit of contemporary wellness, unlocking the transformative potential of Chinese Herbal Medicine for the modern era.

CHAPTER I
Fundamentals of Chinese Medicine

Yin and Yang: Balancing opposing forces

The fundamentals of Chinese medicine revolve around the profound concept of Yin and Yang, a foundational philosophy that permeates every aspect of traditional Chinese healing practices. Yin and Yang, which represent the complementary relationship and interdependence between opposing energies, symbolize the dualistic aspect of reality. This age-old idea, rooted in Taoist philosophy, is essential to comprehend how the body, mind, and cosmos are balanced.

In Chinese medicine, Yin and Yang are conceptualized as two opposite but interrelated forces, each containing the seed of the other. Yang embodies warmth, activity, brightness, and expansion, while Yin encompasses coolness, passivity, darkness, and contraction. For health to be at its best, Yin and Yang must be balanced; any disruption to this equilibrium is said to cause disease.

Within the human body, the organs, tissues, and vital substances are categorized as either Yin or Yang. For instance, the heart and lungs are considered Yang organs, representing activity and movement, while the liver and kidneys are classified as Yin organs, embodying storage and nourishment. The balance between these opposing forces is dynamic, fluctuating in response to external influences, lifestyle, and the natural aging process.

A central tenet of Chinese medicine is the idea that health is a harmonious balance between Yin and Yang. When there is an excess or deficiency of either force, the body falls out of balance, paving the way for illness. To reestablish the balance between Yin and Yang, traditional

Chinese medicine practitioners utilize a range of techniques, such as nutritional treatment, herbal medication, and acupuncture. For example, if a patient is identified as having excess Yang, which manifests as symptoms like restlessness and hot sensations, herbal formulae and dietary changes to support Yin may be prescribed to balance the excess Yang.

The concept of Yin and Yang extends beyond the physical realm to encompass well-being's emotional, mental, and spiritual dimensions. Emotions are classified as Yin or Yang, with anger and excitement representing Yang emotions, while sadness and introspection are associated with Yin. An imbalance in emotional energies can affect the corresponding organ systems, highlighting the interconnectedness of the body-mind-spirit triad in Chinese medicine.

The cyclical nature of Yin and Yang is also reflected in the meridian system, a network of energy pathways through which Qi (vital energy) flows. The meridians are classified as Yin and Yang, each associated with specific organs. The balance of Yin and Yang influences the flow of Qi within these meridians, and disruptions in this flow are believed to underlie various health conditions.

Chinese medicine emphasizes the significance of preventative care and lifestyle alterations to maintain the equilibrium between Yin and Yang and identify and treat abnormalities. Promoting the harmonious flow of vital energy, dietary guidelines, mindful practices, and exercise routines like Qigong and Tai Chi contribute to general well-being.

The Yin and Yang theory impacts larger cosmological and seasonal patterns in Chinese medicine. To enhance health, traditional Chinese medicine practitioners encourage patients to synchronize their activities, nutrition, and way of life with the changing seasons. This is because they acknowledge the natural cycles in the world. As an illustration, winter is seen as a Yin season; during this time, Yin needs to be nurtured by warming foods and enough sleep.

To sum up, the foundations of Chinese medicine—embodied in the idea of Yin and Yang—offer a comprehensive framework for comprehending both health and illness. This ancient therapeutic paradigm is unique due to its integration of physical, emotional, and spiritual dimensions, dynamic balance within the body, and interplay of opposing forces. Through the study of Yin and Yang, practitioners and patients alike set out on a path toward maximum health, guided by the concepts of harmony and balance that have stood the test of time in traditional Chinese medicine.

The Five Elements theory

The Five Elements theory, deeply embedded in the philosophy of traditional Chinese medicine, constitutes a cornerstone in understanding the intricate dynamics of the human body and the universe. Originating from ancient Taoist cosmology, this elemental framework – Wood, Fire, Earth, Metal, and Water – serves as a guiding principle in diagnosing and treating ailments, promoting balance, and illuminating the interplay of energies within and beyond the individual.

The first element, wood, represents expansion, development, and energy. Wood energy, which is associated with spring, conveys the upward surge of fresh life, like the emerging shoots of plants poking through the ground. The smooth flow of Qi, the life-giving force that permeates every part of existence, is attributed to the liver and gallbladder in the human body, which are linked to the Wood element. An excess of Wood energy might show itself as anger, irritation, or digestive problems. The treatment for these imbalances usually consists of techniques to calm and balance the liver.

Following the cyclical order of the seasons and the natural flow of Qi, Fire emerges as the next elemental force. Representing warmth, illumination, and transformation, Fire corresponds to the summer season, a time of peak energy and abundance. In the body, the Fire element is linked to the heart and small intestine, regulating circulation, emotional well-being, and digestion. Imbalances in Fire energy may manifest as symptoms like anxiety, insomnia, or digestive discomfort, prompting interventions focusing on nourishing and harmonizing the heart's Qi.

Summer gives way to late summer, and the Earth element becomes dominant. Earth represents stability, sustenance, and balance and is connected to the stomach and spleen in the human body. These organs are essential for breaking food into nutrient-rich compounds during digestion and assimilation. An imbalance in the energy of Earth might cause weariness, stomach problems, or an unanchored feeling. Interventions in Chinese medicine frequently center on strengthening the Earth element through dietary and lifestyle changes.

Metal, the elemental force associated with autumn, embodies clarity, precision, and discernment qualities. Linked to the lungs and large intestine in the human body, Metal governs respiration, elimination, and the ability to let go. A disruption in Metal energy may manifest as respiratory issues, grief, or constipation. Treatment strategies involve fortifying the Metal element and supporting the lungs' capacity to inspire and release.

Water, the final element in the Five Elements theory, represents the depths of winter – a season of stillness, introspection, and conservation. Corresponding to the kidneys and bladder, Water symbolizes the source of life's essence and the reservoir of vital energy. Imbalances in Water energy may manifest as issues related to the urinary system, fear, or a sense of depletion. Chinese medicine interventions seek to nurture the Water element, emphasizing rest, healing, and the restoration of essential energies during the winter season.

Integral to the Five Elements theory is the concept of the Sheng cycle, or the Generating cycle, which outlines the mutually nourishing relationships between the elements. Wood generates Fire, Fire causes Earth, Earth generates Metal, Metal generates Water, and Water generates Wood. This cycle highlights the dynamic equilibrium that keeps life alive by illuminating the interdependence and connectivity of the elemental forces.

On the other hand, the Ke or Controlling cycles outline the inter-element checks and balances. Wood rules the Earth, which leads the Water, which owns the Fire, which oversees the Metal, which governs the Wood. This cyclical interaction balances the system by preventing any element from becoming overly dominant or insufficient.

The Five Elements theory extends its influence beyond the physical body, providing insights into well-being's emotional, mental, and spiritual dimensions. Each element is associated with specific emotions, virtues, and aspects of consciousness. Understanding these correlations enables traditional Chinese medicine practitioners to offer holistic interventions that address the multifaceted nature of health and balance.

In conclusion, the Five Elements theory in traditional Chinese medicine represents a profound and comprehensive framework for understanding the dynamic interplay of energies within the human body and the natural world. This elemental philosophy guides the diagnosis and treatment of ailments through the cyclical dance of Wood, Fire, Earth, Metal, and Water. It illuminates the intricate connections between well-being's physical, emotional, and spiritual dimensions. As individuals align themselves with the cyclical rhythms of nature and harmonize the elemental forces within, they embark on a journey toward optimal health, balance, and a deeper understanding of the profound wisdom encapsulated in the Five Elements theory.

Qi and Blood: Essential life energies in Chinese medicine

The foundational ideas of traditional Chinese medicine (TCM) are Qi and Blood, which stand for the vital life forces that move through the body to maintain health. These energies provide the basis for understanding the dynamic equilibrium necessary for general well-being. They have their roots in classical Chinese philosophy and are intimately associated with the concepts of Yin and Yang.

Qi is the animating essence that permeates all aspects of existence; it is commonly translated as vital energy or life force. The invisible energy drives internal processes, preserves equilibrium, and moves along a system of meridians to ensure that tissues and organs perform in unison. Qi is more than just energy; it's also awareness, intentionality, and consciousness. According to Traditional Chinese Medicine (TCM), disturbances or imbalances in the flow of Qi are thought to cause various health issues, including emotional and physical disorders.

The concept of Qi is intricately connected to the breath, as breathing is seen as a direct manifestation of the body's absorption of Qi from the surrounding environment. Techniques like Tai Chi and Qigong are meant to develop and harmonize Qi, encouraging its unrestricted movement all over the body. Qi supports healthy health and well-being when it is plentiful and unhindered.

Complementing the notion of Qi is the concept of Blood, which, in TCM, encompasses more than its Western physiological understanding. Blood represents the material manifestation of Qi, containing red and white blood cells and the nutritive essence derived from food and fluids. It circulates through the vessels, providing nourishment to organs and tissues. A robust Blood supply is crucial for maintaining vitality, supporting growth, and ensuring the proper functioning of bodily processes.

The relationship between Qi and Blood is dynamic and interdependent. Qi propels the movement of Blood, while Blood provides the substance and nourishment for Qi. This symbiotic relationship underscores these energies' integral role in TCM, with imbalances in either Qi or Blood seen as potential sources of disharmony and disease.

TCM practitioners assess the quality and quantity of Qi and Blood by considering various factors, including pulse diagnosis, tongue examination, and patient history. A pulse diagnosis, in particular, involves evaluating the characteristics of the radial pulse, providing insights into the state of Qi and Blood in different organ systems. A strong, smooth pulse indicates robust Qi and Blood circulation, while irregularities may show imbalances requiring attention.

Imbalances in Qi and Blood are associated with various health issues in TCM. Deficient Qi may manifest as fatigue, weakness, and susceptibility to illness, while excessive Qi can lead to restlessness and insomnia. Similarly, Blood deficiency may present as a pale complexion, dizziness, or scanty menstruation, while Blood stagnation may result in pain, bruising, or menstrual irregularities.

TCM treatment plans aim to have the blood and qi flowing again in harmony. Dietary advice, lifestyle changes, acupuncture, and herbal treatment are used to treat particular imbalance patterns. More specifically, acupuncture seeks to create balance inside the body by stimulating and controlling the flow of Qi through specific locations along the meridians.

Qi and Blood also play essential functions in the menstrual cycle. For women to experience a regular and healthy menstrual cycle, there must be a smooth flow of Qi and Blood. Qi and Blood imbalances are frequently used to evaluate disorders, including amenorrhea, dysmenorrhea, or irregular menstruation. This helps guide treatment plans to bring the reproductive system back into balance.

In summary, the concepts of Qi and Blood in traditional Chinese medicine provide a profound understanding of the energetic dynamics that underlie health and vitality. These essential life energies, intimately connected to the broader principles of Yin and Yang, form the basis for diagnosis and treatment in TCM. Through the cultivation and harmonization of Qi and Blood, individuals can embark on a journey toward optimal well-being, addressing physical ailments and nurturing the balance of mind, body, and spirit. As the flow of Qi and Blood is restored and maintained, the body's innate capacity for healing and resilience is harnessed, reflecting the timeless wisdom encapsulated in the foundational principles of traditional Chinese medicine.

CHAPTER II
The Role of Chinese Herbs

Understanding the principles of herbal medicine

Understanding the principles of herbal medicine is a journey into the rich tapestry of nature's healing bounty, a realm where the wisdom of traditional practices converges with modern scientific inquiry. Herbal medicine, often referred to as herbalism or phytotherapy, is grounded in the belief that plants possess unique properties capable of promoting health, preventing illness, and restoring balance to the body. This age-old practice is deeply ingrained in cultures worldwide, drawing on various plant species with medicinal properties.

At the core of herbal medicine lies the holistic approach to health, acknowledging the interconnectedness of the body, mind, and spirit. Unlike conventional medicine, which often targets specific symptoms or isolated aspects of health, herbalism embraces the idea that the entire person, their lifestyle, and the underlying causes of imbalance must be considered. The tenets of ancient medicinal systems like Ayurveda, ancient Chinese Medicine, and Native American herbal traditions align with this holistic paradigm. In these systems, plants are seen not only as discrete substances but as living, breathing beings that contain all of life.

Herbal medicine operates on the premise that plants contain many bioactive compounds, each with unique therapeutic properties. These compounds may include alkaloids, flavonoids, essential oils, tannins, and many others, contributing to herbs' diverse array of medicinal actions. The holistic approach extends beyond the biochemical constituents, recognizing the synergy among plant compounds and the complex interplay of these compounds with the human body.

Herbalists employ various methods to extract and administer the medicinal components of plants. These methods include decoctions, infusions, tinctures, poultices, and topical applications. Each process is chosen based on the specific properties of the plant and the desired therapeutic outcome. Decoctions, for instance, involve simmering plant material in water to extract compounds, while tinctures use alcohol or glycerin to capture a broader spectrum of constituents.

A fundamental tenet of herbal medicine is the recognition of individuality in treatment. Herbalists consider not only the presenting symptoms but also each individual's unique constitution, lifestyle, and environmental factors. This personalized approach aligns with constitutional medicine, where an individual's inherent strengths and weaknesses guide the selection of herbs to restore balance. For instance, adaptogenic herbs like Ashwagandha or Ginseng are often recommended to support the body's resilience to stress, adapting their actions based on the individual's specific needs.

Herbal medicine also emphasizes the importance of preventative care and the maintenance of overall well-being. Herbs are not solely reserved for addressing illnesses but are integrated into daily life to promote vitality and resilience. Herbal tonics, for example, are formulations designed to nourish and strengthen specific organ systems, fostering optimal health.

While the holistic principles of herbal medicine remain steadfast, the field has evolved to integrate scientific validation and evidence-based practices. Modern research has delved into the pharmacological actions of plant compounds, elucidating their mechanisms of action and potential applications in various health conditions. This marriage of traditional wisdom and scientific rigor has propelled herbal medicine into complementary and integrative healthcare, garnering recognition and acceptance within conventional medical circles.

Herbal medicine's adaptability is one of its advantages. Plants can offer a spectrum of actions, ranging from anti-inflammatory and antimicrobial to adaptogenic and immune-modulating. For example, Turmeric is celebrated for its anti-inflammatory properties, Echinacea is revered for its immune-boosting effects, and Chamomile is cherished for its calming and digestive benefits. The diversity of plant actions allows herbalists to tailor formulations to address various health concerns.

The principles of herbal medicine also extend beyond individual herbs to the art of formulation. Herbalists skillfully combine multiple herbs to create synergistic blends that enhance efficacy and address the complexities of health conditions. Formulation involves considering each herb's energetics, tastes, and therapeutic actions to create a balanced and effective remedy. This holistic approach to formulation aligns with the understanding that the whole is greater than the sum of its parts.

As individuals navigate the realm of herbal medicine, it becomes evident that empowerment and education are integral components. Herbalists often act as guides, empowering individuals to take an active role in their health by understanding the properties of herbs, making informed choices, and incorporating herbal remedies into their self-care practices. This educational aspect fosters a sense of self-reliance and promotes a deeper connection between individuals and the natural world.

In conclusion, understanding the principles of herbal medicine is an exploration of the profound relationship between humans and the plant kingdom. It is a journey into the art and science of harnessing the healing potential of nature to support health and well-being. Herbal medicine embodies the timeless wisdom of traditional healing practices while evolving to integrate scientific knowledge. As individuals embrace holistic principles, they discover the therapeutic power of plants and embark on a path of self-discovery, sustainability, and a harmonious connection with the natural world.

Classifications of Chinese herbs

The classifications of Chinese herbs form a comprehensive and intricate system that has evolved over centuries, reflecting the nuanced understanding of traditional Chinese medicine (TCM) practitioners. This system categorizes herbs based on their energetic properties, flavors, meridian affiliations, and therapeutic actions. By delving into these classifications, one gains insight into the complex interactions between herbs and their impact on the body's energy and balance.

In TCM, herbs are classified based on their energetic nature, which is associated with the principles of Yin and Yang. Yin herbs are considered cooling and nourishing and are often associated with substances derived from plant roots and leaves. Yang herbs, on the other hand, are warming and invigorating and are often linked to plant parts like seeds and fruits. This classification corresponds with the TCM idea that the body's Yin and Yang energy should be balanced to sustain optimal health.

Another critical aspect of herb classification in TCM is the consideration of flavors, which are believed to have distinct effects on the body's energy. The five flavors – sweet, sour, bitter, salty, and spicy – are associated with specific organ systems and meridians. Sweet flavors are considered nourishing and harmonizing; sour flavors have astringent and consolidating effects; bitter flavors clear heat and drain dampness; salty flavors soften hardness and dissipate accumulations; and spicy flavors disperse Qi and invigorate circulation. The interplay of these flavors in herbal formulations aims to address specific imbalances and promote harmony within the body.

Furthermore, Chinese herbs are classified based on their meridian affiliations, linking them to specific channels through which Qi flows. Each herb is associated with one or more meridians, and its affinity for these energy pathways influences its therapeutic actions. This meridian classification allows practitioners to target specific organ systems and address imbalances in a targeted manner. For example, an herb with an affinity for the liver meridian may be chosen to address conditions related to liver Qi stagnation.

Herbs are also categorized based on their therapeutic actions, encompassing a wide range of bodily effects. These actions include tonifying, reducing, warming, cooling, and moving. Tonifying herbs are used to strengthen and nourish the body, lowering herbs are employed to eliminate excess conditions, warming herbs invigorate and warm the body, cooling herbs clear heat and cool the system, and moving herbs promote the circulation of Qi and blood. The selection of herbs with specific therapeutic actions is tailored to address the unique patterns of imbalance observed in each individual.

Additionally, Chinese herbs are often classified based on their specific functions within herbal formulations. Chief herbs play a primary role in addressing the main pattern of disharmony, deputy herbs support the top herb by reinforcing its actions or addressing secondary patterns, assistant herbs enhance the therapeutic effects of the chief and deputy herbs while mitigating potential side effects, and envoy herbs harmonize the overall formula and guide the actions of the other herbs. This hierarchical classification system allows for creating well-balanced and effective herbal formulations tailored to individual needs.

Understanding the classifications of Chinese herbs is integral to the practice of TCM, where herbal formulations are often tailored to address the unique constitution and patterns of disharmony in each patient. The intricate balance of Yin and Yang, flavors, meridians, therapeutic actions, and functions guide practitioners in creating holistic and personalized herbal prescriptions. This approach exemplifies the holistic philosophy of TCM, where herbs are viewed not as isolated compounds but as dynamic entities working synergistically to restore balance and promote health within the intricate web of the body's energetic system.

In conclusion, the classifications of Chinese herbs represent a sophisticated system that reflects the profound wisdom and holistic approach of traditional Chinese medicine. By considering the energetic properties, flavors, meridians, therapeutic actions, and functions of each herb, TCM practitioners can create nuanced and personalized formulations to address the intricate patterns of disharmony observed in each individual. This method offers a distinctive viewpoint on the art and science of healing within the framework of traditional Chinese medicine, highlighting the close relationship between herbal medicine and the concepts of Yin and Yang.

Methods of preparation and administration

Methods of preparation and administration are crucial facets of utilizing herbs in traditional Chinese medicine (TCM), representing a meticulous and time-honored approach to harnessing the therapeutic properties of botanical substances. TCM recognizes that the efficacy of herbs is not only influenced by their inherent properties but also by the methods used to prepare and administer them. These methods, deeply rooted in ancient practices, have evolved over centuries and play a vital role in ensuring herbal remedies' safety, potency, and tailored application.

One of the primary methods of preparing herbs in TCM is decoction, which involves boiling raw herbs to extract their active constituents. This method is particularly favored for bulk herbs, including roots, barks, twigs, and seeds. Decoctions are often employed when a robust and immediate effect is desired, as the boiling process efficiently extracts water-soluble compounds. The preparation typically involves simmering the herbs in water for an extended period, allowing the release of both volatile and non-volatile constituents. While decoctions are potent and practical, they may pose challenges regarding taste and compliance due to their intense flavors and lengthy preparation time.

In contrast to decoctions, herbal infusions involve steeping herbs in hot water to extract their medicinal properties. This method is commonly used for leaves, flowers, and delicate plant parts. Herbal teas, a popular form of infusion, offer a more palatable alternative to decoctions. Infusions are suitable for herbs with volatile constituents that may be compromised by prolonged exposure to heat. This method is often chosen when a gentler extraction process is preferred or when addressing more subtle imbalances.

Tinctures represent another method of herbal preparation involving the extraction of active compounds using alcohol or glycerin. This method is particularly effective for extracting water-soluble and alcohol-soluble constituents, providing a concentrated and shelf-stable form of herbal medicine. Tinctures offer convenience and portability, making them a practical choice for self-administration. In addition to serving as a preservative, the alcohol base in tinctures prolongs the shelf life of the plant extract. However, dietary constraints or alcohol sensitivity may affect the approach used.

Powdered herbs, obtained by grinding dried plant material, provide a versatile and easily customizable form of herbal medicine. Powders can be encapsulated for convenient consumption or mixed with liquids or food.

Herbs with strong smells or scents benefit from this technique because encapsulation helps to hide these qualities. Additionally, powdered herbs allow for easy dosage adjustments, which makes them appropriate for customized therapy regimens. However, elements like particle size and the possible oxidation of some ingredients may impact powdered herbs' effectiveness.

Topical applications of herbs, such as herbal poultices, salves, or ointments, involve direct contact with the skin to address localized conditions. This technique is frequently used for skin disorders, musculoskeletal problems, and external injuries. Herbal poultices can be applied topically to the diseased area; they are prepared by mixing mashed or powdered herbs with a media such as water or oil. For a topical application or massage, liniments—which are made by distilling the qualities of herbs into alcohol or oil—are frequently utilized.

Extracting herbal properties into alcohol or oil is often used for massage or topical application. The skin, being a semi-permeable barrier, allows for the absorption of certain herbal constituents, offering targeted relief.

In TCM, the preparation method is intrinsically linked to the concept of herbal formulas – combinations of multiple herbs chosen to create a synergistic effect. Herbal formulas are meticulously crafted to address the specific patterns of disharmony observed in an individual. Each herb within a formula plays a distinct role – the chief herb targets the main pattern of disharmony, deputy herbs support and reinforce the top herb, assistant herbs enhance therapeutic effects and mitigate side effects, and envoy herbs harmonize the overall formula.

Administration of herbal formulas is tailored to individual needs and may involve a combination of different methods. Oral administration in decoctions, infusions, tinctures, or powdered herbs is joint for internal conditions. External conditions may be addressed with topical applications such as liniments or poultices. The nature of the situation influences the choice of administration method, the preferences of the patient, and the therapeutic goals.

In conclusion, methods of preparation and administration in traditional Chinese medicine exemplify the precision and individualization inherent in herbal practice. Whether utilizing decoctions, infusions, tinctures, powders, or topical applications, TCM practitioners carefully select methods that align with each herb's unique characteristics and the individual's specific needs. This nuanced approach enhances the efficacy of herbal medicine and ensures that the administration is practical, palatable, and tailored to the diverse conditions encountered in clinical practice. As herbal medicine continues to be integrated into modern healthcare, the wisdom encapsulated in these traditional methods remains a cornerstone in the art and science of botanical healing.

CHAPTER III
Common Chinese Herbs and Their Properties

Exploring popular herbs in Chinese medicine

Exploring popular herbs in Chinese medicine unveils a diverse and time-honored pharmacopeia that has been integral to traditional Chinese medicine (TCM) practice for millennia. These herbs, drawn from various parts of plants, have demonstrated therapeutic efficacy in addressing a broad spectrum of health conditions. Rooted in the principles of balancing Yin and Yang, harmonizing the body's vital energies (Qi), and supporting the various organ systems, these herbs contribute to the holistic approach of TCM. This exploration provides a glimpse into the rich tapestry of popular Chinese herbs, their properties, and the conditions they are traditionally used to address.

Ginseng (Panax ginseng), also called the "king of herbs," is highly valued for its adaptogenic properties, aiding the body's recovery from stress and return to balance. In TCM, it is categorized as a Qi tonic that uplifts the body's life force. Ginseng has long been used to boost immunity, increase general vigor, and improve mental and physical endurance. It is also regarded as a Shen tonic, enhancing mental and spiritual faculties.

Astragalus (Huang Qi): Astragalus is a renowned herb in TCM known for its immune-boosting properties. Classified as a Qi tonic, it strengthens the body's resistance to external pathogens, promotes vitality, and supports the functions of the lungs and spleen. Astragalus is often included in formulations to prevent and recover from respiratory infections.

Licorice Root (Gan Cao): Licorice root is valued for its harmonizing properties in TCM. It is frequently used to moderate the actions of other herbs in a formula and enhance their efficacy. Licorice is also known for its soothing effect on the digestive system, making it a standard inclusion in formulations addressing stomach discomfort and irritability.

Reishi Mushroom (Lingzhi): Reishi is a revered medicinal mushroom in TCM, recognized for its ability to tonify the Qi and nourish the blood. It is often used to support the immune system, alleviate fatigue, and promote a calm and focused mind. Reishi is also considered a Shen tonic, contributing to emotional well-being.

In Traditional Chinese Medicine (TCM), Chinese angelica, also known as Dang Gui (Angelica Sinensis), is vital for blood feeding. It is widely used to treat blood-deficiency disorders, control the menstrual cycle, and relieve menstrual pain. Considered a mild herb, Dang Gui invigorates and harmonizes the blood.

Hawthorn Berry (Shan Zha): Hawthorn berries are employed in TCM for their ability to aid digestion and promote cardiovascular health. They are often included in formulations to alleviate food stagnation and support the movement of Qi in the digestive system. Hawthorn is also valued for its potential to regulate blood circulation.

Chrysanthemum Flower (Ju Hua): Chrysanthemum flowers are known for their cooling properties in TCM. They are commonly used to clear heat from the body, particularly in the eyes. Chrysanthemum tea is a popular beverage in Chinese culture, enjoyed for its refreshing and calming effects.

Schisandra Berry (Wu Wei Zi): Schisandra is categorized as an adaptogenic herb in TCM, known for supporting the body's resilience to stress. It is used to tonify the Qi, nourish the kidneys, and harmonize the various organ systems. Schisandra is often included in formulations designed to enhance vitality and combat fatigue.

Turmeric (Jiang Huang): While not native to China, turmeric has found its way into TCM formulations for its anti-inflammatory and blood-invigorating properties. It is traditionally used to address conditions involving Qi and blood stagnation, such as pain and inflammation.

White Atractylodes (Bai Zhu): White Atractylodes are classified as a Qi tonic in TCM, primarily benefiting the spleen and stomach. It often addresses digestive issues, fatigue, and dampness-related conditions. White Atractylodes are known for their ability to fortify the digestive Qi.

These popular herbs exemplify the diversity and versatility of Chinese herbal medicine, each contributing unique therapeutic actions and properties. It is important to note that the efficacy of these herbs is often realized within the context of a holistic approach, where formulas are carefully crafted to address the individual's specific patterns of disharmony. TCM practitioners leverage the synergy among multiple herbs to create balanced formulations that harmonize the body's energetic pathways and promote overall well-being.

As interest in traditional healing practices grows globally, these popular Chinese herbs have transcended cultural boundaries and gained recognition for their potential health benefits. Modern research continues to explore the pharmacological actions of these herbs, shedding light on their mechanisms of action and potential applications in integrative healthcare.

In conclusion, exploring the world of popular herbs in Chinese medicine provides a glimpse into a sophisticated system of healing that has withstood the test of time. These herbs, celebrated for their holistic approach and ability to address various health concerns, reflect the profound connection between nature and human well-being. As individuals integrate these herbs into their wellness routines, they engage in a tradition that spans centuries, embracing the wisdom of Chinese herbal medicine to support health and harmony in the body, mind, and spirit.

Properties and therapeutic uses of each herb

Understanding each Chinese herb's properties and therapeutic uses is a nuanced journey into the intricate world of traditional Chinese medicine (TCM). Each herb, carefully selected for its specific qualities, contributes to the holistic approach of TCM, aiming to balance the body's vital energies, harmonize organ systems, and address patterns of disharmony. This exploration delves into several refreshing Chinese herbs' properties and therapeutic uses, shedding light on their traditional roles in promoting health and well-being.

Ginseng (Panax ginseng): Ginseng, known as the "king of herbs" in TCM, is revered for its adaptogenic properties. Classified as a Qi tonic, ginseng is traditionally used to strengthen the body's vital energy, enhance physical and mental endurance, and promote overall vitality. Its adaptogenic nature allows it to assist the body in adapting to stress, making it a valuable herb for individuals facing physical or mental challenges. Additionally, ginseng is considered a Shen tonic, supporting cognitive functions and emotional well-being.

Astragalus (Huang Qi): Astragalus is a potent herb classified as a Qi tonic in TCM. Its therapeutic uses revolve around boosting the immune system, strengthening the body's resistance to external pathogens, and promoting overall vitality. Often included in formulations for preventing and recovering from respiratory infections, astragalus is valued for its ability to tonify the Qi and support the functions of the lungs and spleen.

Licorice Root (Gan Cao): Licorice root, known as Gan Cao in TCM, is prized for its harmonizing properties. Licorice enhances their efficacy and mitigates potential side effects when used to moderate the actions of other herbs in a formula. Beyond its role as a harmonizer, licorice root is recognized for its soothing effect on the digestive system, making it a standard inclusion in formulations addressing stomach discomfort, irritability, and digestive issues.

Reishi Mushroom (Lingzhi): Reishi mushrooms hold a special place in TCM as a potent herb for nourishing the Qi and blood. Traditionally used to support the immune system, alleviate fatigue, and promote a calm and focused mind, reishi is considered a Shen tonic, contributing to emotional well-being. Its adaptogenic properties make it a valuable herb for individuals seeking balance in both physical and mental realms.

Dang Gui (Angelica Sinensis): Dang Gui, also known as Chinese Angelica, is a crucial herb in TCM for nourishing the blood. It is widely used to treat blood-deficiency disorders, control the menstrual cycle, and relieve menstrual pain. Dang Gui is a mild herb with blood-harmonizing and blood-invigorating properties; this makes it especially good for women's health.

Hawthorn Berry (Shan Zha): Hawthorn berries play a vital role in TCM, primarily for their effects on digestion and cardiovascular health. Used to alleviate food stagnation and support the movement of Qi in the digestive system, hawthorn berries are valued for their ability to regulate blood circulation. This makes them a standard inclusion in formulations addressing digestion and cardiovascular well-being issues.

Chrysanthemum Flower (Ju Hua): Chrysanthemum flowers, known as Ju Hua in TCM, possess cooling properties and are commonly used to clear heat from the body. This is particularly beneficial for addressing conditions related to excess heat, such as those affecting the eyes. Chrysanthemum tea, made from flowers, is a popular beverage in Chinese culture, celebrated for its refreshing taste and calming effects.

Schisandra Berry (Wu Wei Zi): Schisandra is categorized as an adaptogenic herb in TCM, known for supporting the body's resilience to stress. It is used to tonify the Qi, nourish the kidneys, and harmonize the various organ systems. Schisandra is often included in formulations designed to enhance vitality, combat fatigue, and promote well-being.

Turmeric (Jiang Huang): Although not native to China, turmeric has found its way into TCM formulations for its anti-inflammatory and blood-invigorating properties. Traditionally used to address conditions involving Qi and blood stagnation, such as pain and inflammation, turmeric offers a unique perspective on integrating herbs from diverse cultural traditions.

White Atractylodes (Bai Zhu): White Atractylodes are classified as a Qi tonic in TCM, primarily focusing on benefiting the spleen and stomach. It is often used to address digestive issues, fatigue, and conditions related to dampness. Valued for its ability to fortify the digestive Qi, white atractylodes is a foundational herb in formulations designed to support the digestive system.

Understanding the properties and therapeutic uses of each Chinese herb is central to the practice of TCM, where herbs are often combined in intricate formulations to address the unique disharmony observed in each individual. The selection and synergy of these herbs contribute to the holistic approach of TCM, emphasizing the interconnectedness of the body, mind, and spirit. As individuals explore the world of Chinese herbal medicine, they engage in a tradition that spans centuries, appreciating the wisdom embedded in these botanical treasures that continue to play a vital role in promoting health and balance.

How to incorporate these herbs into daily life

Incorporating Chinese herbs into daily life offers a holistic approach to well-being, embracing the principles of traditional Chinese medicine (TCM) that emphasize balance, harmony, and the interconnectedness of the body, mind, and spirit. Integrating these herbs into daily routines not only honors a rich cultural tradition but also taps into the potential health benefits derived from the wisdom of nature. This exploration delves into practical ways to seamlessly include Chinese herbs in daily life, recognizing the diverse forms these herbs can take and the various aspects of health they may support.

Herbal Teas: One of the most accessible and enjoyable ways to incorporate Chinese herbs into daily life is herbal teas. Traditional Chinese herbal tea blends, readily available in stores or easily crafted at home, offer a delightful and soothing ritual. Herbs like chrysanthemum, goji berries, and dried tangerine peel can be steeped to create aromatic and flavorful teas. These teas provide a moment of relaxation and offer potential benefits for the eyes, immune system, and respiratory health.

Culinary Adventures: Chinese herbs can seamlessly find their way into the kitchen, enriching daily meals with flavor and health benefits. Herbs like astragalus, ginseng, and Chinese yam can be incorporated into soups, stews, and broths, infusing dishes with unique properties. This culinary integration not only enhances the taste of the food but also allows the herbs to contribute to the overall nourishment and support of the body.

Herbal Supplements: For those seeking a convenient and concentrated form of herbal support, herbal supplements are a viable option. These supplements, often available in capsule or tincture form, provide a standardized dosage of specific Chinese herbs. Incorporating herbal supplements into a daily routine allows for a consistent intake of beneficial compounds, promoting long-term well-being and addressing particular health goals.

Essential oils and aromatherapy: Chinese herbs with aromatic qualities, such as eucalyptus, lavender, and mint, can be used. Using critical oils from these herbs, aromatherapy provides a relaxing and uplifting sensory experience.

Herbal Skincare: Chinese herbs have a longstanding tradition of being utilized in skincare formulations for their potential benefits. Incorporating ginseng, goji berries, and licorice root into skincare routines can provide antioxidant properties, promote skin vitality, and address specific skin concerns. Whether infused into facial cleansers, toners, or moisturizers, these herbs contribute to a holistic approach to skincare.

Herbal Infusions in Water: For a refreshing and hydrating option, infusing water with Chinese herbs adds a subtle flavor while offering potential health benefits. Herbs like mint, chrysanthemum, or hawthorn berries can be added to water and left to infuse, creating a naturally flavored beverage. This simple practice encourages adequate hydration and introduces the gentle influence of herbal elements into daily life.

Herbal Rituals: Establishing herbal rituals can infuse daily life with intentional moments of self-care and reflection. Whether through the preparation of herbal teas, the application of herbal skin care products, or the incorporation of aromatherapy, these rituals create a space for mindfulness and connection with the inherent wisdom of nature. This mindful integration fosters a sense of balance and harmony amid daily demands.

Herb Gardening: For those with a green thumb, cultivating a home herb garden can be rewarding.

Growing Chinese herbs like mint, lavender, or cilantro provide a sustainable source for culinary and wellness purposes. Engaging in herb gardening connects individuals with these plants' life cycles and allows for a hands-on approach to incorporating herbs into daily life.

Herbal Meditation: Traditionally, meditation has been linked to specific Chinese herbs, such as frankincense and sandalwood. An atmosphere favorable for rest and reflection can be produced by burning herbal incense or utilizing meditation oils infused with herbs. These herbs improve mental clarity and the sensory experience when added to mindfulness or meditation practices.

In summary, incorporating Chinese herbs into everyday life is a dynamic and adaptable undertaking consistent with the ideas of holistic health. Herbs provide various ways to support well-being, whether savored in teas, recipes, skincare routines, or scented experiences. People can develop a stronger bond with nature and benefit from the extensive history of Chinese herbal medicine by incorporating these activities into their daily routines.

CHAPTER IV
Herbal Formulas and Prescriptions

Combinations of herbs for specific health conditions

Combining Chinese herbs for specific health conditions is a cornerstone of traditional Chinese medicine (TCM), reflecting the holistic approach that addresses the root causes of imbalance rather than merely alleviating symptoms. TCM practitioners carefully select and formulate combinations of herbs based on the individual's unique constitution, patterns of disharmony, and the specific health condition being addressed. The art and science of blending Chinese herbs to produce synergistic effects that support healing and bring the body back into balance is examined in this section.

Respiratory Health: For individuals facing respiratory challenges, TCM often employs a combination of herbs to address symptoms such as cough, congestion, and shortness of breath. Herbs like platycodon (Jie Geng) and apricot seed (Xing Ren) may be combined to clear phlegm and alleviate coughing, while mulberry bark (Sang Bai Pi) is added to promote the resolution of excess lung heat. These combinations aim to harmonize the respiratory system, supporting the lungs and the body's overall energetic balance.

Digestive Disorders: Chinese herbs are frequently combined to address a range of digestive disorders, including indigestion, bloating, and irregular bowel movements. A classic combination might include herbs like ginger (Gan Jiang) and magnolia bark (Hou Po) to harmonize the stomach and relieve nausea. White atractylodes (Bai Zhu) and poria mushroom (Fu Ling) may be added to strengthen the spleen and address dampness, contributing to improved digestive function.

Women's Health: Combinations of Chinese herbs play a crucial role in addressing women's health issues, such as irregular menstruation, hormonal imbalances, and menopausal symptoms. For menstrual irregularities, herbs like Chinese peony root (Bai Shao) and dong quai (Dang Gui) are often combined to nourish the blood and regulate the menstrual cycle. Additionally, combinations for menopausal support may include herbs like Rahmanian (Shu Di Huang) and black cohosh (Sheng Ma) to address hormonal imbalances and alleviate symptoms such as hot flashes.

Immune Support: Chinese herbal combinations strengthen the immune system, particularly during times of increased vulnerability to external pathogens. Renowned herbs like astragalus (Huang Qi) and ligustrum (Nu Zhen Zi) are often combined to tonify the Qi and nourish the immune system. These combinations aim to create a robust defense against illness and promote overall vitality.

Stress and Anxiety: In the realm of mental and emotional well-being, Chinese herbs are combined to address stress, anxiety, and insomnia. Calming herbs like Schisandra (Wu Wei Zi) and Ziziphus seed (Suan Zao Ren) may be blended to soothe the spirit and support restful sleep. These combinations recognize the intricate connection between the mind and body, seeking to restore balance to both aspects of well-being.

Cardiovascular Health: TCM herbal combinations often support cardiovascular health by addressing high blood pressure and poor circulation. Traditional combinations may include herbs like hawthorn berry (Shan Zha) and salvia root (Dan Shen) to promote healthy blood flow, reduce blood pressure, and address patterns of stagnation.

Joint and Muscle Health: Traditional Chinese Medicine (TCM) herbal remedies are intended to relieve pain, lower inflammation, and stimulate blood flow in those suffering from joint and muscle aches. Combining herbs such as white willow bark (Bai Liu) and Eucommia bark (Du Zhong) can strengthen the bones and ligaments and alleviate stagnation and deficient patterns.

Liver Health: Chinese herbs are often combined to support liver health and address conditions such as liver qi stagnation. Bupleurum root (Chai Hu) and white peony root (Bai Shao) are frequently combined to soothe the liver, relieve stress, and regulate the flow of qi. These combinations aim to restore harmony to the liver and prevent the accumulation of stagnant energy.

Kidney Health: In Traditional Chinese Medicine, the kidneys are essential. Herbal formulas are made to tonify kidney essence and treat ailments like exhaustion, lower back pain, and problems with reproduction. Herbs that support lifespan and physical vigor, such as Rehmannia (Shu Di Huang) and deer antler (Lu Jiao Jiao), can be combined to nourish the kidneys.

Allergies: Chinese herbs are combined to address allergies by regulating the immune response and alleviating symptoms such as sneezing and nasal congestion. Combining herbs like magnolia flower (Xin Yi Hua) and schisandra (Wu Wei Zi) may help modulate the body's reaction to allergens and relieve allergic symptoms.

In conclusion, combining Chinese herbs for specific health conditions embodies the holistic philosophy of TCM, recognizing the interconnectedness of bodily systems and the importance of addressing root imbalances. These combinations, tailored to individual needs, showcase traditional Chinese medicine's intricate knowledge and wisdom, offering a personalized and comprehensive approach to health and healing. As individuals explore the world of TCM herbal combinations, they engage in a time-honoured tradition that harmonizes the body, mind, and spirit for optimal well-being.

Creating balanced and tailored herbal formulas

Creating balanced and tailored herbal formulas is a nuanced and intricate process that draws upon centuries of traditional Chinese medicine (TCM) wisdom. This treatment approach is based on the complex relationships between the body's organs, the Yin and Yang concepts, and the Five Elements. The goal of creating a Chinese herbal formula is to address the underlying imbalances and symptoms that give rise to illness, ultimately bringing the body's internal systems back into balance and harmony.

At the core of Chinese herbal medicine is the concept of individualized treatment. Practitioners carefully assess a patient's overall health, considering physical symptoms, emotional well-being, lifestyle, and environmental factors. This holistic approach ensures that the herbal formula is tailored to the specific needs of the individual, acknowledging the unique constitution and imbalances that may be contributing to their health issues.

One fundamental aspect of creating a balanced herbal formula is understanding the Yin and Yang energies within the body. In TCM, health is viewed as a state of dynamic equilibrium between these opposing forces. Imbalances can arise due to excesses or deficiencies in either Yin or Yang, leading to various health issues. Herbal formulas aim to restore this equilibrium by addressing the specific imbalances present in an individual.

The Five components theory improves our knowledge of imbalances by assigning Wood, Fire, Earth, Metal, and Water components to organs and tissues. Every component is linked to particular organs and the functions that go along with them. By examining the interplay among these components, practitioners can discern patterns of discord and choose herbs that specifically address the impacted organs, fostering equilibrium throughout the system.

The process of creating a balanced formula begins with a thorough diagnostic assessment. This may involve examining the patient's tongue, pulse, and overall constitution. Additionally, practitioners inquire about the patient's medical history, lifestyle, and emotional well-being to comprehensively understand the individual's health status.

Once the diagnostic information is gathered, the practitioner selects a combination of herbs that work synergistically to address the identified imbalances. The art of formulation is combining herbs that enhance each other's therapeutic effects while mitigating potential side effects. Some herbs may serve as the principal ingredients, targeting the root cause of the imbalance, while others may support and harmonize the formula, ensuring a holistic approach to healing.

In a Chinese formula, herbs are often categorized into primary, secondary, and sometimes tertiary roles based on their functions. Primary herbs are the main ingredients that target the root cause, secondary herbs support the primary herbs or address accompanying symptoms, and tertiary herbs may be added to adjust the formula to the patient's specific constitution or to counteract potential side effects.

The compatibility of herbs is a critical consideration in Chinese herbal formulations. Certain combinations can enhance the therapeutic effects, while others may lead to undesirable interactions or side effects. Traditional herbalists rely on their extensive knowledge of herb-herb interactions and their understanding of the patient's unique constitution to create a harmonious and effective formula.

In addition to balancing Yin and Yang, herbalists consider the concept of "Jun-Chen-Zuo-Shi" when formulating. This refers to the chief (Jun), assistant (Chen), envoy (Zuo), and guide (Shi) herbs within a formula. The chief herb addresses the primary pattern or condition, the assistant herbs enhance the effects of the top herb or target secondary patterns, the envoy herbs guide the formula to specific meridians or organs, and the guide herbs harmonize the formula and mitigate potential side effects.

Flexibility is another hallmark of Chinese herbal medicine. As a patient's condition evolves, the herbal formula can be adjusted to accommodate changes in symptoms or underlying imbalances. This adaptability allows practitioners to fine-tune the treatment plan over time, ensuring it remains tailored to the individual's dynamic health needs.

When making potent concoctions, the quality and authenticity of the plants are crucial. Chinese herbalists frequently depend on reliable vendors and sources to guarantee the strength and purity of their herbs. The formula's effectiveness is directly impacted by the integrity of the herbs, which is why skilled practitioners go to considerable lengths to source premium ingredients.

To sum up, developing customized and well-balanced Chinese herbal formulae is an intricate procedure rooted in the age-old theories of traditional Chinese medicine. A thorough evaluation of the patient's general health is part of it, along with knowledge of Yin and Yang, the Five Elements, and the expert blending of herbs to treat symptoms and underlying imbalances. Compatibility, in-depth understanding of herbal qualities, and flexibility in formula adaptation as the patient's condition changes are necessary for this formulation. In the end, Chinese herbal medicine seeks to restore balance and harmony to the body's complex systems by providing a comprehensive and individualized approach to healing.

The holistic approach to addressing root causes

The core tenets of traditional Chinese medicine (TCM), which emphasize a thorough understanding of the interrelated systems within the body, are reflected in the holistic approach to treating root problems. According to this holistic viewpoint, the body is seen as an integrated whole in which all organs and systems work together harmoniously. Chinese herbal formulae seek to improve long-term health and restore equilibrium to the body by correcting imbalances at their root.

At the heart of this holistic approach is the concept of the body's vital energy, known as Qi. In TCM philosophy, Qi flows through meridians, nourishing organs and tissues. Imbalances in Qi, whether excess or deficiency, are believed to be at the core of many health conditions. By diagnosing and treating these imbalances, Chinese herbal formulas aim to regulate the flow of Qi, promoting a state of equilibrium and preventing the recurrence of symptoms.

Root causes in Chinese herbal prescriptions are often identified through a comprehensive diagnostic process. TCM practitioners employ various methods, including pulse and tongue examination, questioning about symptoms, medical history, and lifestyle factors. This detailed assessment allows the practitioner to gain insights into the overall state of the patient's health, identifying patterns of disharmony and pinpointing the root causes of their condition.

The holistic approach extends beyond the physical realm, acknowledging the intricate connection between emotions and health. Emotions are considered a significant aspect of TCM diagnosis, and imbalances in emotional well-being are seen as potential contributors to physical ailments.

For instance, chronic stress may lead to Qi stagnation, affecting the proper functioning of organs and meridians. Chinese herbal formulas are, therefore, tailored not only to address physical symptoms but also to rebalance the emotional aspects of an individual's well-being.

The comprehensive approach's examination of environmental impacts and lifestyle factors is another crucial component. Chinese herbal remedies are frequently made to work with lifestyle changes to promote general health and stop imbalances from recurring.

The holistic nature of Chinese herbal medicine is evident in the emphasis on treating the whole person rather than isolated symptoms or conditions. Practitioners recognize that the body is a dynamic and interconnected system, and imbalances in one area can affect the entire organism. For example, a digestive issue may manifest as skin problems, and a skilled TCM practitioner will seek to address the root cause in the digestive system rather than merely treating the skin symptoms.

Chinese herbal formulae address specific disharmony patterns by considering the interconnections between different organs, the Five Elements, and the interplay of Yin and Yang energy. Herbalists who comprehend the underlying imbalances can select herbs that complement each other to address a condition's underlying causes. This method aims to restore equilibrium to the intricate network of interactions within the body beyond the reductionist approach of identifying and treating particular symptoms.

The adaptability of Chinese herbal formulas is a crucial aspect of their holistic nature. As the patient's condition evolves, the prescription can be adjusted to accommodate changes in symptoms or imbalances. This personalized and dynamic approach allows practitioners to refine the treatment plan over time, ensuring it remains tailored to the individual's unique constitution and health journey.

The holistic perspective also extends to the concept of preventive medicine in TCM. Rather than waiting for symptoms to manifest, Chinese herbal medicine emphasizes maintaining balance and preventing imbalances from developing. This proactive approach involves regular patient health assessments, lifestyle counseling, and herbal formulas to support overall well-being.

The quality and authenticity of herbs play a pivotal role in the holistic approach to Chinese herbal medicine. Practitioners prioritize sourcing high-quality herbs from reputable suppliers to ensure the purity and potency of the formulas. The integrity of the herbs directly influences their therapeutic effects and the overall success of the treatment. This commitment to quality reflects the deep respect for the healing properties of plants within the TCM tradition.

In conclusion, the holistic approach to addressing root causes in Chinese herbal formulas and prescriptions embodies the essence of traditional Chinese medicine. To find and address the underlying imbalances causing health problems, practitioners consider the interdependence of environmental, emotional, and physical elements. This method seeks to improve long-term well-being and restore the system to balance rather than just treating symptoms. Chinese herbal medicine offers a holistic worldview that aligns with the dynamic nature of health and healing, emphasizing customized care, flexibility, and preventive tactics.

CHAPTER V
Diagnostic Methods in Chinese Medicine

Traditional diagnostic techniques (tongue diagnosis, pulse reading, etc.)

Traditional Chinese medicine (TCM) relies on a rich tapestry of diagnostic techniques honed over centuries, offering valuable insights into the body's health. Among these, tongue diagnosis and pulse reading stand out as cornerstone methods, playing a pivotal role in assessing the overall balance of the body's vital energies and identifying patterns of disharmony.

Tongue diagnosis in TCM involves meticulously examining the tongue's color, shape, coating, and moisture level. Since the tongue is said to be a reflection of the internal organs, alterations in its appearance might provide essential details about the health of the body. Practitioners pay attention to the tongue's body's color, which reflects the Blood and Yin conditions. A reddish-purple tongue may indicate excess heat, whereas a pale tongue may indicate a blood deficit. The tongue's shape is also essential; anomalies like swelling, fissures, or deviations might point to various imbalances.

The coating on the tongue is closely scrutinized, as it reflects the state of the digestive system and the presence of pathogens. A thin, white coating is considered normal, but thickness, color, or moisture changes can signal imbalances. For example, a thick yellow coating may suggest the presence of heat or dampness, while a dry coating may indicate Yin deficiency. The moisture level of the tongue is associated with the body's hydration and the balance between Yin and Yang.

Pulse reading, another essential diagnostic technique in TCM, involves palpating the radial artery at the wrist. The practitioner assesses the pulse's quality, rhythm, and strength in different positions, corresponding to the twelve primary meridians and organs. In contrast to the predominant focus of Western medicine on heart rate, TCM pulse diagnosis offers a more intricate comprehension of Qi and Blood movement throughout the body.

The pulse is categorized based on depth, speed, width, and strength. Each position and quality of the pulse is associated with specific organs and meridians, allowing practitioners to identify patterns of disharmony. For instance, a wiry or choppy pulse may indicate Liver Qi stagnation, while a weak pulse could suggest Qi deficiency. The simultaneous assessment of multiple pulse positions enables practitioners to understand the patient's internal landscape comprehensively.

In addition to tongue diagnosis and pulse reading, TCM practitioners use other diagnostic methods to gather a holistic understanding of the patient's health. Observation includes assessing the patient's complexion, demeanor, and body movements, offering clues about the state of Qi, Blood, and the overall balance of Yin and Yang. For example, a patient with a pale complexion may be experiencing Blood deficiency, while excessive movement may suggest the presence of internal Wind.

Listening and smelling, the "four pillars" of TCM diagnosis, involve paying attention to the patient's voice, breathing, and distinct odors. Changes in the voice's tone or quality can provide information about the state of the Lungs, while certain odors may indicate the presence of internal heat or dampness. These sensory aspects contribute to the multifaceted diagnostic approach of TCM, allowing practitioners to gather information beyond what is observable through visual and tactile means.

By integrating these diagnostic techniques into TCM, practitioners can identify the root causes of health issues and adjust treatment plans to address imbalances. For example, a patient presenting with digestive problems and a red, swollen tongue with a yellow coating may have Damp-Heat in the digestive tract. The selection of specific herbs and acupuncture points to treat the imbalance will be based on this diagnosis.

One of the strengths of TCM diagnostic techniques is their ability to detect imbalances early, often before symptoms manifest. This proactive approach aligns with the traditional emphasis on preventive medicine, allowing practitioners to address imbalances and promote well-being before developing more significant health issues. The nuanced understanding gained through diagnostic methods enables TCM practitioners to provide personalized and targeted interventions for each individual.

It is essential to note that TCM diagnostic techniques are not isolated; they are interwoven and complement each other to form a comprehensive diagnostic framework. The tongue and pulse readings, in particular, are often used in conjunction to validate findings and refine the diagnosis. For example, a wiry pulse indicating Liver Qi stagnation may be corroborated by a tongue that shows signs of tension or deviation.

Despite the effectiveness of traditional diagnostic techniques, TCM practitioners recognize the importance of integrating modern medical assessments when necessary. These may involve imaging studies, laboratory testing, and consultations with other medical specialists to guarantee a comprehensive picture of the patient's health situation. Integrating contemporary and conventional methods enables a more thorough and patient-focused approach to treatment.

In conclusion, traditional diagnostic techniques in Chinese medicine, such as tongue diagnosis and pulse reading, form the bedrock of a holistic and personalized approach to healthcare. These methods, deeply rooted in ancient wisdom, offer practitioners valuable insights into the body's internal balance, guiding the selection of appropriate interventions. By combining visual, tactile, and sensory observations, TCM practitioners can identify patterns of disharmony, often at an early stage, and address the root causes of health issues. Integrating traditional diagnostic methods with modern assessments further enhances the efficacy and comprehensiveness of healthcare practices, reflecting the adaptability and relevance of traditional Chinese medicine in the contemporary world.

Understanding the body's signs and symptoms

Understanding the body's signs and symptoms through Chinese diagnostic methods is a profound and intricate process deeply embedded in traditional Chinese medicine (TCM) philosophy. This approach transcends the conventional model of isolating symptoms and instead seeks to unravel the underlying patterns of disharmony within the body. TCM practitioners interpret the body's signals as a reflection of the dynamic interplay between Yin and Yang energies, the flow of Qi (vital energy), and the balance of the body's internal organs.

One of the primary diagnostic methods in TCM is tongue diagnosis, where practitioners meticulously examine the tongue's color, shape, coating, and moisture. The tongue is regarded as a mirror of the body's internal organs, and variations in its appearance offer valuable insights. For instance, a pale tongue may indicate Blood deficiency, while a red or purplish hue may suggest excess heat. Changes in the tongue's coating, such as thickness, color, or moisture level, provide additional information about the digestive system and the presence of pathogens. A skilled practitioner can discern the body's overall condition by synthesizing these various tongue characteristics.

Pulse reading is another indispensable diagnostic tool in TCM, involving palpating the radial artery at the wrist. Unlike Western medicine, which primarily focuses on heart rate, TCM pulse diagnosis delves into the nuances of pulse quality, rhythm, and strength at different positions corresponding to the twelve primary meridians and organs. Each pulse quality and position is associated with specific organ systems, allowing practitioners to identify patterns of disharmony. For example, a wiry or choppy pulse may indicate Liver Qi stagnation, while a weak pulse could suggest Qi deficiency. Integrating information from multiple pulse positions enables practitioners to construct a comprehensive and nuanced understanding of the patient's internal landscape.

Observational diagnostics, encompassing aspects such as complexion, demeanor, and body movements, play a crucial role in TCM diagnosis. Practitioners keenly observe a patient's external appearance, looking for signs of imbalance in the complexion, such as paleness, redness, or a yellowish tint. Changes in body movements, such as excessive restlessness or sluggishness, provide further insights into the state of Qi and Blood. Facial expressions, body language, and overall demeanor contribute to the practitioner's understanding of the patient's emotional well-being, a vital aspect in TCM diagnosis where emotions are considered integral to overall health. Listening and smelling, considered the "four pillars" of TCM diagnosis, involve paying attention to the patient's voice, breathing, and distinct odors. Changes in the tone or quality of the voice offer clues about the state of the Lungs, while certain odors may indicate the presence of internal heat or dampness. These sensory aspects contribute to the multifaceted diagnostic approach of

TCM, allowing practitioners to gather information beyond what is observable through visual and tactile means.

Instead of being seen as distinct occurrences, TCM views the body's indications and symptoms as interconnected expressions of the body's overall homeostasis. For instance, disharmony patterns such as blood scarcity, stagnant liver qi, or extreme heat might result in headaches. By recognizing these patterns, TCM practitioners can create customized treatments that address the root causes of symptoms and bring the body's equilibrium back to normal.

A crucial aspect of TCM diagnostics is the recognition of patterns rather than the mere identification of individual symptoms. Symptoms are manifestations of deeper imbalances, and TCM practitioners aim to identify the pattern or syndrome underlying a set of symptoms. This approach allows for a more nuanced and targeted treatment strategy, addressing not only the immediate discomfort but also the root cause of the disharmony. The holistic nature of TCM diagnostics is evident in its ability to consider the interplay between the body's physical, emotional, and environmental aspects. Emotions are considered integral to health, and imbalances in emotional well-being are recognized as potential contributors to physical ailments. For example, chronic stress may lead to Qi stagnation, affecting the proper functioning of organs and meridians. TCM diagnostics, therefore, encompass an exploration of the patient's emotional landscape to gain a comprehensive understanding of their overall health.

Understanding the body's signs and symptoms through Chinese diagnostic methods extends beyond the identification of disease and emphasizes the concept of preventive medicine. TCM practitioners aim to detect imbalances at an early stage, often before symptoms manifest, allowing for proactive interventions. By addressing imbalances and promoting overall well-being, TCM aligns with the traditional emphasis on preventing illness and maintaining harmony within the body.

In conclusion, understanding the body's signs and symptoms through Chinese diagnostic methods embodies traditional Chinese medicine's holistic and intricate nature. Tongue diagnosis, pulse reading, observational diagnostics, and sensory assessments provide a comprehensive framework for interpreting the body's expressions of imbalance. Grounded in ancient principles, TCM diagnostics transcends the reductionist view of symptoms and seeks to identify patterns of disharmony, allowing for personalized and targeted interventions. Because environmental, emotional, and physical factors are interdependent, TCM approaches health and healing holistically. It aims to bring the body back into balance and harmony as a dynamic, interconnected organism.

Customizing herbal treatments based on individual assessments

Customizing herbal treatments based on individual assessments through diagnostic methods is a hallmark of traditional Chinese medicine (TCM), reflecting its patient-centered and holistic approach to healthcare. TCM practitioners employ many diagnostic techniques, including tongue diagnosis, pulse reading, and observational assessments, to gain profound insights into each individual's unique constitution and imbalances. These diagnostic methods provide a comprehensive understanding of the body's state of health, allowing practitioners to tailor herbal treatments that address the specific root causes of a patient's condition.

One of the essential diagnostic tools in customizing herbal treatments is tongue diagnosis. By meticulously examining the tongue's color, shape, coating, and moisture, practitioners gain valuable information about the patient's internal balance. For instance, a red or purplish hue on the tongue may indicate excess heat, while a pale tongue may suggest Blood deficiency. Changes in the coating, such as thickness, color, or moisture level, further guide the practitioner in identifying patterns of disharmony related to the digestive system and the presence of pathogens. This detailed analysis forms the foundation for selecting herbs targeting the identified imbalances.

Pulse reading, another essential diagnostic method, provides additional nuances for customizing herbal treatments. By palpating the radial artery at different positions corresponding to the twelve primary meridians and organs, practitioners discern the pulse's quality, rhythm, and strength. Each pulse quality and position is associated with specific organ systems, aiding in the identification of patterns of disharmony. For instance, a wiry or choppy pulse may suggest Liver Qi stagnation, while a weak pulse could indicate Qi deficiency. Integrating information from various pulse positions allows practitioners to create a tailored and nuanced herbal prescription.

Observational diagnostics, encompassing aspects such as complexion, demeanor, and body movements, contribute further to the individualized assessment. Practitioners keenly observe external signs, such as changes in complexion, which may indicate imbalances in Blood, Qi, or specific organ systems. Body movements and overall demeanor provide insights into the state of Qi and emotional well-being. By synthesizing these observations with tongue and pulse readings, practitioners develop a holistic understanding of the patient, allowing for the customization of herbal treatments that address their health's physical and emotional aspects.

Customizing herbal treatments in TCM extends beyond addressing symptoms to target the underlying patterns of disharmony. Symptoms are manifestations of deeper imbalances, and TCM practitioners aim to identify the specific pattern or syndrome underlying a set of symptoms. For example, a patient presenting with digestive issues and a red, swollen tongue with a yellow coating may be diagnosed with Damp-Heat in the digestive system. The herbal treatment is then customized to address this specific pattern, with herbs chosen to clear heat, resolve dampness, and harmonize the digestive system.

The traditional theories of Yin and Yang, the Five Elements, and the meridian system form the basis of the customized approach to TCM herbal treatments. These fundamental ideas offer a framework for comprehending every person's individual constitution and imbalances. To relieve symptoms and restore the body's homeostasis, the goal is to treat the underlying reasons for the disharmony. For example, a patient with Yin and Qi insufficiency symptoms, such as fatigue and a peeling, red tongue, would be recommended a herbal formula to strengthen Qi and nourish Yin.

Flexibility and adaptability are crucial aspects of customizing herbal treatments in TCM. As a patient's condition evolves, the herbal formula can be adjusted to accommodate changes in symptoms or imbalances. This dynamic approach ensures that the treatment remains tailored to the individual's growing health needs. The adaptability of TCM herbal treatments reflects the acknowledgment of the body as a dynamic and interconnected system where imbalances may shift over time.

Another essential consideration in customizing herbal treatments is the compatibility of herbs within a formula. TCM herbalists carefully select herbs that work synergistically to enhance therapeutic effects while mitigating potential side effects. Traditional herbal knowledge guides the compatibility of herbs, ensuring a harmonious blend that addresses the specific imbalances identified through diagnostic methods. For example, a chief herb may target the primary pattern or condition. In contrast, assistant herbs support and enhance the effects, envoy herbs guide the formula to specific meridians or organs and guide herbs harmonize and mitigate potential side effects.

The quality and authenticity of herbs are paramount in customizing TCM herbal treatments. Practitioners rely on trusted sources and suppliers to ensure the purity and potency of their herbs. The herbs' integrity directly influences the formula's efficacy, and experienced practitioners take great care in sourcing high-quality ingredients. This commitment to quality reflects the profound respect for the healing properties of plants within the TCM tradition.

In conclusion, customizing herbal treatments based on individual assessments through diagnostic methods is a cornerstone of traditional Chinese medicine. The meticulous analysis of the tongue, pulse, and observational aspects allows practitioners to gain profound insights into each individual's unique constitution and imbalances. By tailoring herbal treatments to address the specific root causes identified through diagnostic methods, TCM practitioners provide personalized and effective interventions. The individualized approach, rooted in ancient principles and guided by flexibility and adaptability, reflects the holistic nature of TCM and its commitment to restoring balance and promoting well-being in a dynamic and interconnected system.

CHAPTER VI
Chinese Herbal Medicine in Practice

Integrating Chinese herbs into a holistic wellness routine

Incorporating Chinese herbs into a comprehensive wellness regimen embodies the fundamental concepts of traditional Chinese medicine (TCM). It signifies a harmonious marriage of conventional wisdom and contemporary wellness techniques. Thanks to their long history and wide range of medicinal benefits, Chinese herbs are quickly included in holistic health regimens to improve overall well-being, resolve imbalances, and promote balance. This integration is a deliberate and customized approach that considers the person's constitution, health objectives, and the dynamic interaction of environmental, psychological, and physical elements.

Integrating Chinese herbs into a holistic wellness regimen is based on the understanding that the body is a dynamic, linked organism. In traditional Chinese medicine, optimal organ function, a harmonious flow of Qi (vital energy), and a balance of Yin and Yang energies indicate good health. Chinese herbs are selected for their distinct properties and functions; they are intended to alleviate symptoms, treat the root causes of imbalances, and bring the body back into balance. This holistic perspective, which highlights the connections between various aspects of health, aligns well with the broader holistic wellness philosophy.

One of the key benefits of incorporating Chinese herbs into a holistic wellness routine lies in their adaptability and versatility. These herbs are not viewed as isolated remedies for specific ailments but as components of comprehensive formulas designed to address the multifaceted nature of health. Whether targeting digestive issues, stress management, or immune support, Chinese herbal formulas are crafted to consider the intricate relationships between different organ systems and the individual's overall constitution. This adaptability allows individuals to tailor their herbal regimen to their unique health needs and goals, fostering a holistic approach beyond symptom management.

Integrating Chinese herbs into a holistic wellness routine often begins with a comprehensive assessment by a qualified TCM practitioner. Through diagnostic methods such as tongue diagnosis, pulse reading, and observational assessments, the practitioner gains insights into the individual's patterns of disharmony, constitution, and overall health status. This personalized approach ensures that the herbal regimen aligns with the individual's needs, addressing root causes and promoting overall well-being. The practitioner's guidance is invaluable in navigating the vast array of Chinese herbs and selecting the most effective and appropriate for the individual's health goals.

In a holistic wellness routine, Chinese herbs are not considered part of a broader framework encompassing lifestyle factors, dietary choices, and mindful practices. Holistic wellness emphasizes the integration of physical, mental, and emotional well-being, and Chinese herbs complement this integration. For example, a formula tailored to address stress and promote relaxation may complement mindfulness practices such as meditation or yoga, creating a synergistic approach to holistic wellness.

The adaptogenic properties of many Chinese herbs contribute to their effectiveness in promoting resilience and adaptability in the face of stressors. Adaptogens help the body respond more effectively to physical, emotional, or environmental stressors. Herbs such as Ginseng,

Rhodiola, and Astragalus are renowned for their adaptogenic properties, helping the body maintain balance during times of increased demand. By integrating these herbs into a holistic wellness routine, individuals can enhance their capacity to navigate the challenges of modern life while fostering a state of overall well-being.

Digestive health is another crucial aspect of integrating Chinese herbs into holistic wellness. TCM recognizes the importance of a well-functioning digestive system in maintaining overall health, and various herbs are selected to support digestion, absorption, and elimination. For individuals seeking to optimize their digestive wellness, herbal formulas may include ingredients like Hawthorn, Atractylodes, and Licorice, tailored to their specific digestive patterns identified through TCM diagnostic methods.

Integrating Chinese herbs into holistic wellness extends to immune support, an area of increasing importance in today's health-conscious society. Herbs such as Astragalus, Reishi mushroom, and Schisandra are valued for their immune-modulating properties, helping the body maintain a robust defense against external pathogens. This proactive approach aligns with the holistic wellness philosophy of preventing illness and promoting overall resilience rather than reacting to symptoms.

Furthermore, Chinese herbs are often included in beauty and skin care regimens as they address imbalances that may manifest in the skin's appearance. Herbs like Dang Gui and Schisandra are known for their blood-nourishing properties, promoting a radiant complexion and supporting overall skin health. This integrative approach recognizes the connection between internal balance and external manifestations, acknowledging that true beauty arises from a harmonious state of health.

Quality and authenticity are paramount in integrating Chinese herbs into a holistic wellness routine. Individuals are encouraged to source herbs from reputable suppliers and consult with qualified practitioners to ensure the purity and potency of the herbs they incorporate into their routine. This commitment to quality aligns with the broader principles of holistic wellness, emphasizing a conscious and mindful approach to self-care.

In conclusion, integrating Chinese herbs into a holistic wellness routine embodies a synergistic and integrative approach to health. Based on traditional Chinese medicine's tenets, this integration considers the patient's constitution, treats imbalances at the source, and promotes general health. Chinese herbs are versatile and adaptive, making them a good fit within the larger framework of holistic wellbeing, which includes dietary choices, mindful practices, and lifestyle considerations. Chinese herbs can be used for various purposes, such as immune system support, stress relief, digestive health, and skincare. This holistic approach acknowledges the interdependence of mental, emotional, and physical health. Including Chinese herbs in a comprehensive wellness regimen embodies an age-old wisdom still relevant in pursuing optimum health and vitality.

Collaboration with Chinese medicine practitioners

Collaboration with Chinese medicine practitioners represents a synergistic and integrative approach to healthcare that draws upon the ancient wisdom of traditional Chinese medicine (TCM) and the broader framework of modern medical practices. Chinese medicine practitioners, often trained in disciplines such as acupuncture, herbal medicine, and TCM diagnostics, bring a unique perspective to holistic healthcare. The collaboration between Western medicine and Chinese medicine acknowledges the strengths of both traditions, fostering a more comprehensive understanding of health and well-being.

One of the critical areas of collaboration involves TCM diagnostics, which includes tongue diagnosis, pulse reading, and observational assessments. While Western medicine emphasizes laboratory tests and imaging studies, TCM diagnostics offer a complementary approach by providing insights into the body's patterns of disharmony, constitution, and overall health status. Collaborative efforts between Western healthcare professionals and Chinese medicine practitioners allow for a more nuanced and holistic patient understanding, facilitating personalized and targeted interventions.

One of the mainstays of Chinese medicine, acupuncture, is frequently included in team-based healthcare models. It is said that by inserting tiny needles into particular acupuncture spots, Qi (vital energy) flow can be regulated, and the body's equilibrium is enhanced. Acupuncture may be used with traditional therapies for stress reduction, pain management, or supportive care during specific medical procedures. Together, Western and Chinese medicine practitioners provide a more comprehensive approach to patient care by addressing fundamental imbalances and symptom relief.

Another essential component of traditional Chinese medicine is herbal medicine, which provides a wide range of natural treatments made from plants, minerals, and animal products. Working with Chinese medicine practitioners enables the integration of herbal remedies into a patient's care plan, taking into account their patterns of disharmony and constitution. For instance, a cooperative approach combining Western medical procedures and Chinese herbal formulae designed to address side effects, strengthen immune function, and improve overall well-being may benefit cancer therapy patients.

Collaborative initiatives in women's health frequently combine TCM viewpoints with Western gynecological techniques. Chinese medicine has a long history of treating menopausal symptoms, irregular menstruation, and fertility troubles in women. Chinese medicine viewpoints can be incorporated into a thorough treatment plan by working with Western medical professionals. This provides a holistic approach to women's healthcare, including physical and energetic components.

Psychological well-being is another area where collaboration between Western and Chinese medicine practitioners is increasingly recognized. Chinese medicine acknowledges the intricate connection between emotions and physical health, and practices such as acupuncture and herbal medicine can be incorporated to support mental health. Collaborative approaches may involve combining psychotherapy with acupuncture for stress reduction and anxiety management or as a complementary intervention in the treatment of mood disorders.

Integrating traditional Chinese medicine into supportive cancer care is a notable example of successful collaboration. In addition to chemotherapy and radiation therapy, acupuncture and herbal medicine are frequently used to treat side symptoms such as pain, exhaustion, and nausea. Chinese medicine treats patients holistically, promoting not only the physical symptoms but also the mental and energetic health of the patient. Collaborating to treat cancer demonstrates the potential for a comprehensive, patient-focused approach that capitalizes on the strengths of both medical specialties.

While collaboration between Western and Chinese medicine practitioners offers numerous benefits, effective communication, and mutual respect are essential for successful integrative care. Shared decision-making, where both practitioners contribute their expertise and insights, ensures patients receive a well-rounded and tailored approach to their healthcare. Educational initiatives that foster understanding between practitioners of different traditions contribute to a collaborative environment where diverse perspectives are valued.

Collaboration between Western and Chinese medicine practitioners has shown promise in treating chronic pain. Working with Western medical specialists enables acupuncture to be incorporated into pain management regimens. Combining acupuncture with traditional methods like physical therapy and medicine can lead to better pain management and increased patient function.

Globally, traditional Chinese medicine is becoming more and more accepted and integrated into mainstream healthcare systems. Sometimes integrative medicine departments have been developed by hospitals and other medical facilities, bringing together practitioners from various backgrounds, such as Western and Chinese medicine. This collaborative approach recognizes the importance of both the holistic tenets of traditional Chinese medicine and the evidence-based practices of Western medicine while providing patients with various therapeutic options.

In conclusion, collaboration with Chinese medicine practitioners represents a dynamic and inclusive approach to healthcare that combines traditional Chinese medicine's strengths with Western medicine's advancements. The synergy between these two medical traditions enhances treatment options and contributes to a broader understanding of health that embraces the individual's physical and energetic aspects. As collaboration continues to evolve, it holds the potential to shape a future where diverse medical traditions work together synergistically for the benefit of patient-centered care.

Case studies illustrating successful herbal treatments

Case studies serve as compelling narratives that illustrate the successful application of herbal treatments within traditional Chinese medicine (TCM). These real-life examples showcase the efficacy of Chinese herbal medicine in addressing a diverse range of health issues, providing insights into the diagnostic process, treatment strategies, and positive outcomes for patients.

In a case involving a middle-aged woman experiencing chronic fatigue and insomnia, TCM diagnostic methods they played a pivotal role in guiding successful herbal treatments. The practitioner conducted a thorough assessment, including tongue diagnosis and pulse reading, revealing signs of Qi deficiency and Blood stagnation. The herbal formula prescribed included Ginseng to tonify Qi and Dong Quai to invigorate Blood circulation. After several weeks of herbal treatment, the patient reported significant improvements in energy levels and sleep quality, demonstrating the effectiveness of addressing the underlying imbalances identified through TCM diagnostics.

Another illustrative case involves a middle-aged man suffering from recurrent migraines and digestive issues. TCM diagnostic methods, including tongue diagnosis, revealed signs of Liver Qi stagnation and dampness affecting the digestive system. The herbal treatment plan incorporated Chai Hu to soothe Liver Qi and Hou Po to resolve dampness.

In the context of women's health, a case study involving a woman with irregular menstrual cycles and fertility concerns showcases the effectiveness of Chinese herbal treatments. TCM diagnostics identified patterns of Blood deficiency and Liver Qi stagnation. The prescribed herbal formula included herbs like Dang Gui to nourish Blood and Bupleurum to soothe Liver Qi. Following several months of herbal treatment, the patient experienced regular menstrual cycles and successfully conceived, underscoring the role of Chinese herbs in promoting reproductive health.

A case of inflammatory skin conditions, such as eczema or psoriasis, provides insights into the successful integration of herbal treatments. TCM diagnostics, including tongue diagnosis and assessment of the patient's overall constitution, revealed patterns of heat and dampness in the body. The herbal formula incorporated herbs with cooling and detoxifying properties, such as Huang Qin and Zi Cao. Over time, the patient observed a significant reduction in skin inflammation and irritation, emphasizing the ability of Chinese herbs to address skin conditions by targeting underlying imbalances.

A notable case study involves the successful management of stress and anxiety using Chinese herbal medicine—a young professional presented with symptoms of excessive stress, palpitations, and insomnia. TCM diagnostics identified patterns of Liver Qi stagnation and Heart Yin deficiency. The herbal formula included Bai Shao to nourish Liver Blood and Suan Zao Ren to calm the Shen (spirit). The patient reported a notable reduction in stress levels and improved sleep quality, highlighting the efficacy of Chinese herbal treatments in addressing emotional well-being.

In the context of digestive health, a case study featuring a patient with irritable bowel syndrome (IBS) exemplifies the benefits of herbal treatments. TCM diagnostics revealed patterns of spleen deficiency and dampness in the digestive system. The herbal formula incorporated herbs such as Chen Pi to regulate Qi and Bai Zhu and strengthen the Spleen. The patient reported a significant reduction in IBS symptoms, including bloating and irregular bowel movements, showcasing the targeted approach of Chinese herbal medicine in addressing digestive imbalances.

Furthermore, cases involving chronic pain conditions illustrate the successful integration of acupuncture and Chinese herbal treatments. A patient with persistent lower back pain underwent a collaborative approach, combining acupuncture sessions with herbal formulas tailored to address patterns of Kidney deficiency and Qi stagnation.

In conclusion, these case studies provide compelling evidence of the successful application of Chinese herbal treatments across various health conditions. The holistic approach of traditional Chinese medicine, guided by thorough diagnostic methods, allows practitioners to tailor herbal formulas to each individual's unique disharmony patterns. The positive outcomes observed in these cases underscore the versatility and effectiveness of Chinese herbal medicine in promoting health and well-being. As these narratives demonstrate, integrating Chinese herbal treatments into patient care plans contributes to a more comprehensive and personalized approach to healthcare.

CHAPTER VII
Herbal Medicine for Modern Ailments

Addressing common health issues with Chinese herbs

Using Chinese herbs to treat common health problems incorporates the age-old wisdom of traditional Chinese medicine (TCM), providing a customized and all-encompassing approach to well-being. One prevalent health concern that Chinese herbs effectively target is stress and anxiety. Herbs like Bai Shao (White Peony) and Suan Zao Ren (Sour Jujube Seed) are commonly used to nourish the Liver, soothe Liver Qi stagnation, and calm the Shen (spirit). This combination addresses the energetic imbalances associated with stress, promoting emotional resilience and a sense of calm. By considering the interconnectedness of the body and mind, Chinese herbs provide a unique avenue for managing stress beyond symptom suppression.

Digestive issues, including bloating, indigestion, and irregular bowel movements, are frequently addressed with Chinese herbal treatments. Herbs such as Chen Pi (Tangerine Peel) and Bai Zhu (White Atractylodes) are employed to regulate Qi, strengthen the Spleen, and resolve dampness in the digestive system. This comprehensive approach considers the dynamic interplay of the body's energy and the impact on digestive function. Chinese herbs improve gastrointestinal health and overall well-being by restoring harmony to the digestive system.

Chinese herbs are widely used in women's health to address menstrual irregularities, fertility concerns, and menopausal symptoms. Herbs like Dang Gui (Chinese Angelica Root) are renowned for nourishing Blood and regulating the menstrual cycle. For fertility support, herbal formulations may include ingredients such as Shu Di Huang (Rehmannia) and Gui Ban (Turtle Shell), targeting both Yin and Yang aspects of reproductive health. During menopause, herbs like Huang Qi (Astragalus) and Sheng Mai San are employed to tonify and nourish Yin, alleviating symptoms such as hot flashes and mood swings. The holistic approach of Chinese herbs to women's health recognizes the cyclical nature of the female body and aims to restore balance to support overall reproductive well-being.

Chinese herbs are also crucial for treating inflammatory skin diseases like psoriasis and eczema. Herbs with cooling and detoxifying properties, such as Huang Qin (Scutellaria) and Zi Cao (Lithospermum), are combined to address patterns of heat and dampness in the body. This targeted approach alleviates skin inflammation and aims to resolve the underlying imbalances contributing to these conditions. By addressing both the symptomatic and root causes, Chinese herbs provide a holistic solution for individuals struggling with skin-related issues.

In respiratory health, Chinese herbs address common concerns such as coughs, colds, and allergies. Herbs like Ma Huang (Ephedra) and Zi Wan (Purple Aster Root) are utilized to disperse Wind-Cold or Wind-Heat, relieving respiratory symptoms. These herbs also aim to support the body's immune response and strengthen the respiratory system. The adaptability of Chinese herbal formulations allows practitioners to tailor treatments based on the specific nature of respiratory issues, providing a personalized and practical approach to respiratory health.

Herbs from the Chinese pharmacopeia are frequently utilized to manage chronic pain conditions. For instance, formulas containing herbs like Yan Hu Suo (Corydalis Yanhusuo) and Wei Ling Xian (Clematis Root) are designed to invigorate Blood circulation, dispel stasis, and alleviate pain. Whether the pain is associated with musculoskeletal issues or chronic conditions, Chinese herbs provide a holistic and targeted approach to pain management. This comprehensive strategy not only addresses pain symptoms but also works towards restoring balance within the body to prevent the recurrence of discomfort.

Herbs like white attractylodes (Bai Zhu) and patchouli (Huo Xiang) balance Qi, balance the stomach and alleviate moisture. Chinese herbs provide a comprehensive and individualized approach to gastrointestinal health by addressing the underlying patterns of disharmony. Herbal formulations' adaptability makes it possible to customize therapies according to the unique patterns seen in each individual, enhancing the efficacy of these interventions.

Cardiovascular health is another area where Chinese herbs play a supportive role. Herbs like Dan Shen (Salvia) and Shan Zha (Hawthorn) are commonly employed to invigorate Blood circulation, regulate Qi, and support cardiovascular function. This approach addresses specific cardiovascular concerns and considers the broader energetic balance within the body. By promoting optimal circulation and addressing underlying imbalances, Chinese herbs holistically contribute to cardiovascular well-being.

The immune system is known to benefit from Chinese herbal therapy, especially during seasonal changes or exposure to infections. Herbs that tonify Qi and strengthen the body's defense energy include Huang Qi (Astragalus) and Bai Zhu (White Atractylodes). This proactive strategy is in line with traditional Chinese medicine's beliefs, which strongly emphasize the need to keep the immune system strong to fend against illness. Individuals can take a preventative and holistic approach to their health by incorporating immune-supportive herbs into wellness routines.

Furthermore, Chinese herbs are commonly integrated into weight management strategies. Herbs such as He Ye (Lotus Leaf) and Fu Ling (Poria) regulate digestion, promote the elimination of dampness, and support metabolic function. These herbs work in synergy to address weight management's physical and energetic aspects, contributing to a holistic approach that considers individual constitution and imbalances.

In conclusion, addressing common health issues with Chinese herbs represents a holistic and personalized approach to well-being. The versatility of Chinese herbal formulations allows practitioners to tailor treatments based on individual patterns of disharmony, contributing to the effectiveness of these interventions. By considering the interconnectedness of the body's energy, Chinese herbs offer solutions beyond symptom management, aiming to restore balance and promote overall health. As individuals increasingly seek holistic and integrative approaches to health, Chinese herbal medicine plays a valuable and influential role in addressing many common health concerns.

Stress, insomnia, digestive problems, and more

Stress, insomnia, digestive problems, and many other health issues are commonly addressed through the holistic and personalized approach of traditional Chinese medicine (TCM), leveraging the diverse therapeutic properties of Chinese herbs. Stress, often considered a modern epidemic, finds a nuanced solution in the principles of TCM. Chinese herbs such as Bai Shao (White Peony) and Suan Zao Ren (Sour Jujube Seed) are employed to nourish the Liver, soothe Liver Qi stagnation, and calm the Shen (spirit). By addressing the energetic imbalances associated with stress, these herbs provide symptomatic relief and work towards restoring emotional resilience and a sense of calm, emphasizing the interconnectedness of emotional and physical well-being.

Insomnia, a prevalent concern in our fast-paced society, is effectively tackled with Chinese herbal treatments that focus on rebalancing the body's internal energies. Herbs like Huang Lian (Coptis) and Wu Wei Zi (Schisandra) regulate the Heart and Liver, addressing Yin and Yang disharmony patterns. This comprehensive approach acknowledges the role of the heart in sleep regulation and the importance of calming the mind for restful sleep. Chinese herbal formulas for insomnia are tailored to individual patterns, considering factors such as excess or deficiency, further showcasing the adaptability of TCM in providing personalized solutions for sleep disorders.

Digestive problems, encompassing issues like bloating, indigestion, and irregular bowel movements, are effectively managed through the holistic lens of TCM. Herbal formulations such as Bao He Wan, containing herbs like Shen Qu (Massa Fermentata) and Lai Fu Zi (Radish Seed), aim to regulate Qi, harmonize the Stomach, and resolve dampness. This method emphasizes the significance of treating the underlying patterns of disharmony in the digestive system and the symptoms, acknowledging the complex relationship between the stomach and the Spleen. Chinese herbs enhance general well-being and gastrointestinal health by reestablishing equilibrium.

Women's health concerns, ranging from menstrual irregularities to fertility issues and menopausal symptoms, find a supportive ally in Chinese herbal medicine. Herbs like Dang Gui (Chinese Angelica Root) are revered for their ability to nourish Blood and regulate the menstrual cycle. For fertility support, formulations may include ingredients such as Shu Di Huang (Rehmannia) and Gui Ban (Turtle Shell), addressing both Yin and Yang aspects of reproductive health. Chinese herbal medicine's holistic approach to women's health acknowledges the cyclical nature of the female body and offers complete, individualized treatments for different phases of life.

Chinese herbal therapy uses a tailored strategy to treat inflammatory skin disorders, including psoriasis and eczema. To address patterns of heat and dampness in the body, herbs with cooling and detoxifying qualities, like Huang Qin (Scutellaria) and Zi Cao (Lithospermum), are mixed. Chinese herbs completely remedy people with inflammatory skin conditions by addressing symptoms and underlying causes. This holistic approach reduces skin inflammation and addresses the underlying imbalances causing these conditions.

Respiratory health concerns, including coughs, colds, and allergies, are effectively managed through Chinese herbal formulations that aim to disperse Wind-Cold or Wind-Heat. Herbs like Ma Huang (Ephedra) and Zi Wan (Purple Aster Root) address respiratory symptoms and support immune function. The adaptability of Chinese herbal treatments allows for personalized approaches based on the specific nature of respiratory issues, contributing to effective and tailored interventions for individuals seeking respiratory health support.

Chronic pain conditions, a pervasive challenge for many individuals, are addressed with the integrative approach of acupuncture and Chinese herbal medicine. Herbal formulations containing Yan Hu Suo (Corydalis Yanhusuo) and Wei Ling Xian (Clematis Root) are designed to invigorate Blood circulation, dispel stasis, and alleviate pain. Whether the pain is associated with musculoskeletal issues or chronic conditions, the combination of acupuncture and herbal medicine provides a holistic and targeted approach to pain management. This comprehensive strategy not only addresses pain symptoms but also works towards restoring balance within the body to prevent the recurrence of discomfort.

Chinese herbal therapy efficiently treats gastrointestinal problems, from gastritis to irritable bowel syndrome (IBS), by addressing moisture and regulating Qi. Herbs that balance the stomach and control digestion include Huo Xiang (Patchouli) and Bai Zhu (White Attractylodes). Chinese herbs provide a comprehensive and individualized approach to gastrointestinal health by addressing the underlying patterns of disharmony. The versatility of herbal formulations makes it possible to customize treatments according to particular patterns seen in each patient, which increases the efficacy of these interventions.

Cardiovascular health is one of the most important aspects of general health, and Chinese herbs can help maintain good heart function. Herbs used to promote cardiovascular health, regulate Qi, and energize blood circulation include Dan Shen (Salvia) and Shan Zha (Hawthorn). This technique considers the body's overall energy balance while addressing specific cardiovascular issues. Chinese herbs support cardiovascular health by correcting underlying imbalances and encouraging healthy circulation.

A key component of preventative healthcare is immune support, which is why Chinese herbs are often included in wellness regimens. Herbs that tonify Qi and strengthen the body's defense energy include Huang Qi (Astragalus) and Bai Zhu (White Atractylodes). This proactive strategy is in line with traditional Chinese medicine's beliefs, which strongly emphasize the need to keep the immune system strong to fend against illness. People can adopt a preventive and comprehensive approach to their health by including immune-stimulating herbs in everyday practices.

Chinese herbs are part of complete solutions that address weight management's physical and energetic components, which is a complex issue. Herbs that enhance metabolic activity, encourage moisture removal, and regulate digestion include He Ye (lotus leaf) and Fu Ling (Poria). Together, these herbs can help with both the physical elements of managing weight and any underlying energy imbalances that may be causing issues with weight. Chinese herbal formulations are highly customizable, enabling customized methods based on unique constitutions and imbalances.

In conclusion, stress, insomnia, digestive problems, and other health issues find effective and holistic solutions through the diverse therapeutic properties of Chinese herbs. The personalized and adaptable nature of traditional Chinese medicine allows for targeted interventions that address the symptoms and the underlying patterns of disharmony within the body. As individuals increasingly seek holistic and integrative approaches to health, Chinese herbal medicine remains a valuable and influential modality emphasizing the interconnectedness of physical, emotional, and energetic well-being.

The adaptogenic nature of many Chinese herbs

The adaptogenic nature of many Chinese herbs represents a cornerstone of traditional Chinese medicine (TCM), embodying the philosophy of promoting resilience and balance within the body. Adaptogens help the body adapt to stressors and maintain homeostasis, supporting overall well-being. In Chinese herbal medicine, numerous herbs are recognized for their adaptogenic properties, providing a holistic approach to health that addresses the dynamic interplay of internal and external factors.

Ginseng, one of the most renowned adaptogenic herbs in Chinese medicine, exemplifies the concept of adaptability. Famous for its ability to tonify Qi (vital energy) and nourish the Spleen and Lung meridians, Ginseng is often prescribed to enhance physical and mental endurance, combat fatigue, and promote overall vitality. Its adaptogenic nature allows it to modulate the body's response to stress, supporting energy production during periods of increased demand while promoting a sense of calm during emotional stress.

Another well-known adaptogen in Chinese herbal medicine, Rhodiola, has become famous for its capacity to increase resistance to various stressors. Rhodiola is frequently used to enhance cardiovascular health and increase endurance because of its adaptogenic effects on the circulatory system. This adaptogenic herb is thought to influence the release of stress hormones and supports a balanced physiological state, modulating the body's stress response. Rhodiola contributes to TCM's adaptogenic qualities by regulating Qi and bolstering the Kidneys.

Astragalus, a staple in Chinese herbal formulations, is valued for its immune-modulating and adaptogenic effects. This herb is traditionally used to tonify Qi, especially in chronic fatigue and immune deficiency cases. Astragalus's adaptogenic nature enhances the body's ability to resist external pathogens and cope with environmental stressors. By supporting the body's overall vitality, Astragalus exemplifies the adaptogenic principles of TCM that focus on preventing illness and maintaining balance.

In Chinese medicine, Schisandra berry is recognized for its unique combination of five flavors—sweet, sour, salty, bitter, and spicy—and its adaptogenic properties. This herb supports the body's adaptation to stress, improves mental clarity, and enhances physical endurance. Schisandra is often utilized to tonify the Kidneys and Liver, contributing to its adaptogenic effects on physical and emotional well-being.

Holy Basil, known as Tulsi in Ayurvedic medicine and considered an adaptogen in traditional Chinese medicine, is revered for its ability to balance the body's stress response. It is said that holy basil lowers cortisol, eases the symptoms of stress, and encourages serenity. Its adaptogenic effects on respiratory and digestive health are attributed to its frequent association with the Lung and Spleen meridians in Traditional Chinese Medicine.

Many Chinese herbs have adaptogenic properties consistent with the holistic tenets of traditional Chinese medicine, which emphasize the interdependence of different organ systems and the significance of preserving homeostasis within the body. Herbs with a sweet taste, such as licorice root, are prized for their ability to balance various meridians and organ systems. In herbal formulae, licorice is frequently added to balance out the effects of other herbs, improve their effectiveness, and reduce their actions.

In stress management, Chinese herbal formulas often combine adaptogenic herbs to address the multifaceted nature of stress. For instance, a formula may include Ginseng to boost energy and resilience, Rhodiola to improve endurance, and Schisandra to support mental clarity. This synergistic approach reflects the adaptogenic principles of TCM, aiming to alleviate symptoms and enhance the body's overall ability to adapt and maintain balance.

The adaptogenic nature of Chinese herbs is also evident in their application to support the body during times of change, such as seasonal transitions. Herbal formulas designed for seasonal wellness often include adaptogens like Astragalus to strengthen the immune system and enhance the body's ability to adapt to seasonal stressors. This preventative strategy emphasizes the need to preserve balance to fend against illness and advance good well-being, which is consistent with the core ideas of TCM.

Moreover, adaptogenic herbs are frequently integrated into formulations targeting specific organ systems. For example, herbs like Reishi mushroom, revered as the "Mushroom of Immortality," are known for their adaptogenic effects on the immune system and the Liver. Reishi is believed to modulate the immune response, reduce inflammation, and promote liver detoxification. This adaptogenic approach aligns with the holistic perspective of TCM, recognizing the interconnectedness of different organ systems in maintaining overall health.

In conclusion, traditional Chinese medicine's fundamental ideas are reflected in the adaptogenic properties of numerous Chinese herbs, which highlight the body's capacity to adjust to stimuli and preserve equilibrium. Herbs recognized for their adaptogenic qualities include ginseng, rhodiola, astragalus, schizandra, holy basil, licorice, and reishi mushrooms. These adaptogens are incorporated into holistic herbal formulations that consider the individual's constitution and support total well-being, whether the focus is on immune support, stress management, or exhaustion. Chinese herbs are still an excellent resource for building resilience, energy, and balance in the body since people are becoming increasingly interested in holistic approaches to health.

CHAPTER VIII
The Art of Herbal Healing

The connection between mind, body, and herbs

This holistic system recognizes the intricate interplay between mental, emotional, and physical aspects of well-being. In TCM, the mind and body are viewed as interconnected, each influencing the other in a dynamic dance of energy and vitality. Herbs, as essential components of TCM, play a profound role in nourishing this connection, offering therapeutic benefits beyond alleviating physical symptoms to addressing the root causes of imbalance.

Central to the TCM philosophy is the concept of Qi, often translated as vital energy. Qi flows through meridians, which are energetic pathways that connect various organ systems. The mind, embodying consciousness and emotions, is intricately linked to this flow of Qi. Emotional imbalances, such as stress, anxiety, or sadness, are seen as disruptions in the smooth circulation of Qi. Herbs are employed not only to address physical symptoms but also to regulate the flow of Qi and restore harmony to the mind.

Herbs with adaptogenic properties exemplify the intimate connection between the mind and body in TCM. Adaptogens, such as Ginseng and Rhodiola, are believed to modulate the body's response to stress and promote balance or homeostasis. By supporting the body's ability to adapt to stressors, these herbs simultaneously influence the mind, fostering resilience and emotional well-being. The adaptogenic nature of these herbs reflects the holistic approach of TCM, acknowledging the inseparable link between mental and physical health.

The mind-body connection is further underscored by the use of herbs to address conditions with both physical and emotional components. Herbs like St. John's Wort, for instance, are used to reduce anxiety and depression symptoms since mental and physical health are intimately related. According to TCM, the emotional condition is a reflection of the energy system of the body's balance or imbalance, and medicines are used to treat both.

The concept of Shen, often translated as spirit or consciousness, is integral to understanding the connection between mind and body in TCM. Herbs nourish Shen to calm the mind, enhance mental clarity, and support emotional well-being. For instance, herbs like Bai Zi Ren (Arborvitae Seed) and Yuan Zhi (Polygala Root) are traditionally used to soothe the spirit and promote restful sleep. This holistic approach recognizes that a calm and balanced mind is essential for overall health and vitality. In

the context of stress management, the mind-body connection is paramount. Chronic stress not only manifests physically but also profoundly impacts mental and emotional well-being. Because of their adaptogenic qualities, herbs like holy basil reduce stress and encourage mental clarity and serenity. These herbs provide a comprehensive approach to resolving the complicated relationship between stress and psychological and physical health issues associated with contemporary lives.

Herbs to enhance memory and cognitive function is another example of the mind-body link in action. Herbs that nourish the mind, increase blood flow to the brain, and improve mental performance include gotu kola and ginkgo biloba. This method aligns with the TCM viewpoint, which acknowledges the mind's impact on physical vitality and sees mental health as a crucial component of overall well-being.

Herbs are crucial in addressing sleep disorders, emphasizing the intimate relationship between the mind and sleep quality. Herbs like Valerian root and Passionflower are employed to calm the mind, alleviate anxiety, and promote restful sleep. TCM recognizes that sleep is a physical therapeutic process and a time when the mind undergoes essential rejuvenation. Herbs tailored to support the mind-body connection during sleep contribute to overall vitality and well-being.

The mind-body connection is deeply embedded in TCM diagnostic methods, including tongue diagnosis and pulse reading. These diagnostic tools provide insights into physical imbalances and the state of the mind and emotions. For instance, a red tongue with a yellow coating may indicate excess heat in the body, which could be associated with heightened emotions such as anger or frustration. Herbs chosen based on such diagnostic insights aim to rebalance both the physical and emotional aspects, highlighting the inseparable link between the mind and body in TCM.

The concept of the Five Elements in TCM further illustrates the interconnectedness of the mind, body, and herbs. Each element—Wood, Fire, Earth, Metal, and Water—is associated with specific organs, emotions, and physical manifestations. Herbs are chosen to address imbalances within these elements, considering the physical symptoms and the emotional landscape. This holistic approach recognizes that restoring balance within the Five Elements contributes to overall mind and body harmony.

In traditional Chinese medicine, herbs that affect the liver, such as bupleurum and chai hui, are prime examples of the mind-body link. The Liver is linked to feelings like rage and impatience as well as the easy movement of Qi. Emotional imbalances and physical symptoms can occur when the liver's function is impaired. The choice of herbs to support liver detoxification considers these interrelated factors, fostering physical health and dynamic balance.

In conclusion, the connection between mind, body, and herbs is fundamental in traditional Chinese medicine. Herbs are viewed not merely as agents to alleviate symptoms but as potent tools to nourish the entire being, recognizing the inseparable link between mental, emotional, and physical aspects of health. The holistic approach of TCM, deeply rooted in ancient wisdom, emphasizes the importance of balance and harmony within the mind and body, providing a comprehensive framework for promoting overall well-being. As individuals increasingly seek integrative and holistic approaches to health, the profound connection between mind, body, and herbs continues to be a guiding principle in traditional Chinese medicine.

Cultivating a mindful approach to herbal medicine

Cultivating a mindful approach to herbal medicine is essential to embracing the holistic philosophy inherent in traditional healing practices. Mindfulness, rooted in ancient wisdom and increasingly recognized in modern integrative medicine, involves a conscious and focused awareness of the present moment. In the context of herbal medicine, mindfulness extends beyond herbs' physical properties to encompass a deep understanding of their energetic qualities, the unique needs of individuals, and the dynamic interplay between the mind and body.

At the heart of a mindful approach to herbal medicine is recognizing that herbs are not just isolated substances with specific effects but complex expressions of nature's wisdom. Each herb embodies unique flavors, energies, and affinities for different organ systems. Practitioners and individuals alike are encouraged to approach herbal medicine with reverence and appreciation for the inherent intelligence in botanical remedies. By cultivating mindfulness, one can establish a more profound and harmonious integration of herbal medicine into daily life and a stronger connection to the healing powers of herbs.

Mindfulness in herbal medicine involves a keen observation of the body's signals, an awareness of individual constitutions, and a recognition of the interconnectedness of physical, mental, and emotional well-being. For instance, when selecting herbs to address a specific health concern, a mindful approach considers the symptoms and underlying patterns of imbalance within the body. This nuanced understanding allows for customizing herbal formulations tailored to an individual's unique constitution and health goals.

Mindfulness also plays a crucial role in preparing and consuming herbal remedies. Whether brewing a cup of herbal tea or preparing a tincture, engaging with the herbs becomes a meditative practice. This mindful preparation fosters a deeper connection to the healing process and encourages individuals to be present in the ritual of taking herbs. Such awareness extends to the sensory experience – the herbal remedy's taste, aroma, and texture – creating a holistic engagement beyond the medicinal properties alone.

In the mindful exploration of herbal energetics, individuals become attuned to balance within the body. Traditional Chinese Medicine, for instance, classifies herbs based on their energetic properties, such as warming or cooling, and their affinities for specific meridians or organs. A mindful approach involves understanding this energetics and applying them to restore balance. For instance, in addressing a condition characterized by excess heat, a practitioner may choose cooling herbs to harmonize the body's energetic landscape. This attentiveness to herbal energetics contributes to a more holistic and personalized approach to wellness.

Mindfulness extends to the ethical considerations of herbal medicine, encouraging individuals to source herbs responsibly and sustainably. The mindful cultivation and harvesting of herbs emphasize the importance of reciprocity with nature. This ecological awareness aligns with the principles of traditional herbalism, which recognizes the interconnectedness between human health and the planet's health. By mindfully choosing herbs, individuals contribute to preserving biodiversity and the sustainability of herbal resources, fostering a sense of stewardship for the Earth.

In the application of herbal medicine, a mindful approach recognizes the dynamic nature of health and the importance of adaptability. The body's needs may evolve, influenced by seasonal changes, life stages, and external stressors. Practitioners and individuals are encouraged to observe and adjust herbal protocols accordingly, acknowledging that health is dynamic and ever-changing. This adaptability reflects the essence of mindfulness, embracing the present moment and responding to the body's unique requirements with a compassionate and flexible approach.

Mindfulness in herbal medicine also involves an awareness of the mind-body connection and the impact of emotional well-being on overall health. Stress, anxiety, and other emotional factors contribute to patterns of imbalance within the body. Mindful herbalists consider the dynamic landscape when crafting formulations, selecting herbs that address physical symptoms and support emotional resilience. This integrated approach acknowledges the link between mental and physical health, fostering a more comprehensive and effective healing process.

Integrating mindful practices from other traditions, such as meditation and breathwork, further enriches a cautious approach to herbal medicine. These practices enhance self-awareness, promote relaxation, and create a receptive state for the healing properties of herbs. Mindfulness meditation, in particular, has been demonstrated to lower stress, boost general well-being, and increase the effectiveness of holistic health approaches. Including mindfulness practices in daily life can work in conjunction with herbs to promote health and healing synergistically.

Herbal medicine practitioners are not the only ones who should cultivate a mindful attitude; anyone looking to improve their health and well-being should also go on this road. By encouraging people to take an active role in their healing, mindfulness helps them feel empowered and accountable for their well-being. People can make educated decisions, better understand their health, and include herbal medicines in a lifestyle that promotes general vitality and balance by cultivating a mindful relationship with herbs.

In conclusion, a mindful approach to herbal medicine transcends the mere consumption of botanical remedies. It involves a deep engagement with the inherent wisdom of herbs, an awareness of individual needs, and a recognition of the interconnectedness between mind, body, and the natural world. By embracing mindfulness in selecting, preparing, and applying herbs, individuals and practitioners foster a holistic and harmonious relationship with herbal medicine. This mindful approach contributes not only to personal well-being but also to a broader sense of ecological responsibility and a deeper connection to the healing forces of nature.

Herbal rituals and practices for overall well-being

Herbal rituals and practices for overall well-being encapsulate a profound connection between humanity and the healing power of nature, drawing upon the ancient wisdom embedded in traditional herbalism. These rituals, rooted in diverse cultural traditions, are not merely routines but sacred acts that honor plants' innate intelligence and ability to support holistic health. One such ritual involves the preparation of herbal teas, where the infusion of plant essences becomes a ceremonial act. This practice is not only a sensory experience, with the aroma and taste of the herbs engaging the senses, but it also serves as a mindful moment of self-care. Whether it be chamomile's calming effects, peppermint's refreshing qualities, or holy basil's adaptogenic properties, each herbal tea blend becomes a tailored elixir that nurtures both the body and the spirit.

Additionally, incorporating herbal baths into one's routine exemplifies a time-honoured practice that promotes relaxation and rejuvenation. Drawing on the therapeutic qualities of herbs like lavender, calendula, or chamomile, these baths become immersive experiences that transcend the physical act of cleansing. The warmth of the water, coupled with the aromatic herbal infusions, creates a harmonious synergy that not only cleanses the body but also calms the mind. This ritualistic approach acknowledges the importance of mental well-being, intertwining the physical and emotional realms to pursue overall health.

Smudging rituals, often associated with the burning of sage or other aromatic herbs, have been employed by various cultures for centuries to clear negative energy and invite positive influences. This herbal practice, rooted in traditions such as Native American smudging ceremonies, symbolizes a purification process that extends beyond the physical space to include the mind and spirit. The aromatic smoke is believed to carry away stagnant energy, leaving a revitalized environment and a sense of clarity. Incorporating smudging into a wellness routine aligns with the holistic philosophy that overall well-being encompasses the body and the energetic and spiritual dimensions of one's being.

Herbal practices for overall well-being extend into skincare, where botanical ingredients have been cherished for their therapeutic properties. Crafting herbal-infused oils, salves, or creams becomes a ritualistic endeavor, transcending conventional skincare routines. Ingredients such as calendula, comfrey, or lavender are carefully selected for their skin-nourishing qualities, reflecting a holistic understanding that what we apply to our skin can influence our health and overall well-being. This intentional approach to skincare recognizes the skin as a reflection of internal vitality and the gateway through which herbs can positively impact the body.

Herbal rituals also unfold in the form of seasonal wellness practices, aligning with nature's cyclical patterns. Traditional practices, such as the Ayurvedic approach to seasonal cleansing or the Chinese medicine concept of adapting to the energies of each season, involve the strategic use of herbs to support the body's natural rhythms. For example, in the transition from winter to spring, herbs like dandelion and nettle may be incorporated to gently cleanse and invigorate the body after the stagnation of colder months. These seasonal rituals acknowledge the dynamic nature of well-being, recognizing that the body's needs shift with changing environmental influences.

In mindfulness and meditation, herbal practices are supportive companions on the journey to inner peace and self-discovery. Herbal teas, specifically chosen for their calming properties, become integral to meditation rituals. Chamomile, Passionflower, or lemon balm, known for their soothing effects on the nervous system, create a tranquil backdrop for contemplation. Sipping herbal tea becomes a meditative process, grounding individuals in the present moment and enhancing the overall experience of inner stillness.

Gardening itself is a therapeutic herbal practice, inviting individuals to cultivate a connection with the Earth and actively participate in the life cycles of plants. Engaging with herbs from seed to harvest fosters a sense of stewardship and deepens one's appreciation for the vitality inherent in nature. The act of growing herbs becomes a reciprocal relationship, where individuals not only benefit from the plants but also contribute to their well-being through mindful cultivation practices. This hands-on approach aligns with the belief that overall well-being is intricately tied to our relationship with the natural world.

Herbal rituals extend into the culinary realm, where using herbs in cooking transforms meal preparation into a nourishing practice. Beyond flavor enhancement, herbs like rosemary, thyme, and oregano bring their medicinal properties to the dining table. This culinary alchemy aligns with the ancient wisdom that views food as medicine, recognizing that the herbs we incorporate into our diets contribute to our overall health. Infusing meals with various herbs becomes a culinary celebration of well-being, intertwining the pleasure of eating with the intentional consumption of medicinal plants.

Moreover, the creation of herbal tinctures embodies a ritualistic approach to harnessing the potent qualities of plants. The process of steeping herbs in alcohol or glycerin, allowing them to macerate over time, transforms the herbal constituents into concentrated elixirs. This intentional extraction method reflects a deep respect for the alchemical process and the desire to capture the essence of herbs for therapeutic use. Incorporating herbal tinctures into daily routines becomes a self-care ritual, offering a convenient and potent means of integrating herbal support into one's overall wellness strategy.

In the broader community and social well-being context, herbal rituals can take the form of collective ceremonies or gatherings. Traditional practices like tea ceremonies, where individuals come together to share and appreciate herbal infusions, foster a sense of community and interconnectedness. These shared experiences promote the physical benefits of herbal consumption and contribute to the emotional and social dimensions of overall well-being. Communicating over herbal beverages becomes a celebration of health and unity, transcending individual well-being to encompass the collective spirit. In

conclusion, herbal rituals and practices for overall well-being encapsulate a rich tapestry of traditions, each weaving a unique connection between individuals and the healing power of plants. From mindful tea ceremonies to the intentional crafting of herbal skincare, each ritual reflects a conscious engagement with nature's bounty and recognizes the profound interconnectedness between mind, body, and the natural world. These herbal practices are not isolated routines but sacred acts that honor the wisdom of ancient traditions and offer a pathway to holistic well-being. As individuals increasingly seek integrative and mindful approaches to health, these herbal rituals stand as timeless guides, inviting us to embrace the transformative power of plants in our journey toward overall well-being.

CHAPTER IX
Sustainability and Ethical Considerations

Responsible sourcing of Chinese herbs

Responsible sourcing of Chinese herbs is critical to ensuring ethical, sustainable, and high-quality herbal medicine practices. With its rich tradition of herbal medicine spanning thousands of years, China supplies a significant portion of the world's medicinal herbs. As the demand for traditional Chinese herbs grows globally, the importance of responsible sourcing practices becomes increasingly apparent. Ethical considerations in the sourcing process encompass ecological sustainability, fair labor practices, cultural preservation, and the quality and safety of harvested herbs.

One primary concern in the responsible sourcing of Chinese herbs is the impact on biodiversity and the environment. Many traditional Chinese herbs are wildcrafted or grown in their native habitats. Irresponsible harvesting practices, driven by high demand, can lead to overharvesting and depletion of natural resources. To address this, responsible sourcing initiatives promote sustainable harvesting methods, cultivation practices, and the preservation of biodiversity. Cultivating medicinal herbs that respect natural ecosystems, promote regenerative agriculture, and minimize environmental impact is crucial for the long-term health of herbal traditions and the ecosystems from which these herbs are derived.

Fair labor practices are another crucial aspect of responsible sourcing. Many Chinese herbs are hand-harvested, requiring a significant amount of manual labor. Ensuring that the individuals involved in herb cultivation and harvesting are treated ethically and receive fair compensation is essential for creating a sustainable supply chain. Responsible sourcing initiatives emphasize transparency in the supply chain, traceability of herbs from cultivation to distribution, and adherence to fair labor standards. Responsible sourcing aims to create a more equitable and socially responsible industry by prioritizing the well-being of those involved in the herbal trade.

Preserving cultural practices and knowledge is integral to the responsible sourcing of Chinese herbs. Traditional Chinese medicine (TCM) has deep roots in Chinese culture, and many herbs are deeply intertwined with local customs and traditions. The responsible sourcing Chinese herbs involves working collaboratively with local communities, respecting indigenous knowledge, and acknowledging the cultural significance of herbal practices. This approach ensures the preservation of valuable cultural heritage and fosters a sense of community empowerment as local practitioners and communities become stewards of their herbal traditions.

Quality and safety are paramount considerations in the responsible sourcing of Chinese herbs. The global herbal market is susceptible to adulteration, contamination, and misidentification of plant species. Responsible sourcing initiatives prioritize quality control measures to address these concerns, including rigorous testing for authenticity, purity, and absence of contaminants. Collaboration between herbal suppliers, growers, and regulatory bodies ensures that Chinese herbs meet established quality standards and comply with safety regulations. By emphasizing quality assurance, responsible sourcing safeguards the integrity of herbal medicine and promotes consumer confidence in the safety and efficacy of herbal products.

Certification programs play a significant role in promoting responsible sourcing practices for Chinese herbs. Organizations such as the Good Agricultural and Collection Practices (GACP) and Good Manufacturing Practices (GMP) have developed standards and guidelines for cultivating, harvesting and processing medicinal plants, including Chinese herbs. These certifications provide a framework for responsible sourcing, addressing ecological, social, and quality considerations.

Engaging in direct relationships with herb growers and suppliers is a crucial strategy for responsible sourcing. Building transparent and collaborative partnerships fosters a deeper understanding of the entire supply chain, from cultivation to distribution. This direct engagement allows for open communication, shared knowledge, and the establishment of mutually beneficial relationships. By working closely with herb producers, responsible sourcing practices support local economies, encourage sustainable cultivation methods, and strengthen the overall resilience of the herbal supply chain.

Education and awareness initiatives are essential components of responsible sourcing of Chinese herbs. Creating awareness among consumers, practitioners, and industry stakeholders about the importance of responsible sourcing practices fosters a demand for ethically produced herbs. Educational efforts can include information about sustainable harvesting, fair labor practices, and the cultural significance of herbal traditions. By empowering individuals with knowledge, responsible sourcing initiatives seek to shape consumer choices, encourage ethical business practices, and contribute to the broader movement toward a more sustainable and accountable herbal industry.

In conclusion, the responsible sourcing Chinese herbs is a multifaceted endeavor that addresses ecological, social, cultural, and quality considerations. Responsible sourcing initiatives contribute to the long-term viability and integrity of the herbal medicine industry by promoting sustainable harvesting, fair labor practices, cultural preservation, and adherence to quality standards. A rising number of people worldwide are becoming interested in traditional Chinese medicine and herbal medicines, highlighting the significance of ethical sourcing techniques. The moral and ecological practices adopted in the responsible sourcing of Chinese herbs protect biodiversity and the planet's natural resources while preserving the cultural legacy and general well-being of the communities that practice the ancient art of herbal healing.

Environmental impact and conservation efforts

The environmental impact of various human activities, including the sourcing and production of herbal products, has become a growing concern in the context of global sustainability. Traditional herbal medicine, deeply rooted in nature and reliant on diverse plant species, is not exempt from these considerations. The harvesting, cultivating, and processing of herbs for medicinal use can have significant ecological consequences if not managed responsibly. As awareness of environmental issues continues to rise, the herbal industry is increasingly recognizing the importance of conservation efforts to mitigate its impact on ecosystems, biodiversity, and the planet's overall health.

Harvesting practices, particularly wildcrafted herbs, can have profound implications for plant populations and ecosystems. Overharvesting, driven by escalating demand for herbal products, threatens the sustainability of certain plant species. This issue is especially pertinent in regions where traditional herbs are endemic or play a crucial role in local ecosystems. Conservation efforts seek to solve these issues by encouraging sustainable harvesting methods that consider plant population regeneration rates, respect harvesting quotas, and integrate ethical wildcrafting principles. Sustainable methods maintain the delicate balance between human use and the protection of plant species by ensuring that the harvest of herbs does not surpass the natural capacity of ecosystems to renew.

How herbal medicine is cultivated also has a significant impact on the environment. Applying pesticides indiscriminately, using synthetic fertilizers, and large-scale monoculture can all lead to pollution, biodiversity loss, and soil degradation. Conservation-oriented cultivation methods are becoming more popular in the herbal sector as a reaction to these worries. Conservation efforts within the herbal industry support the restoration of soil health, preservation of water resources, and general resilience of agricultural ecosystems by coordinating herbal cultivation with environmental sustainability principles. Agroecological approaches, such as polyculture and organic farming, prioritize soil health, foster biodiversity, and minimize the use of synthetic inputs.

One of the main goals of environmental initiatives in the herbal sector is biodiversity conservation. The richness of Earth's ecosystems is reflected in the diversity of plant species employed in traditional herbal medicine. Many plant species, some of which have unique therapeutic qualities, are threatened by habitat loss and overexploitation. Conservation efforts highlight the value of maintaining biodiversity by safeguarding natural areas, assisting in reintroducing threatened species and promoting the sustainable use of wildcrafted plants. In addition to helping to conserve biodiversity, initiatives to identify and highlight lesser-known plant species with therapeutic potential also help to preserve critical genetic resources and traditional knowledge for subsequent generations.

The impact of herb cultivation on water resources is another crucial consideration within conservation efforts. Conventional agriculture practices, including herb cultivation, can contribute to water pollution through synthetic fertilizers and pesticide runoff. Additionally, large-scale irrigation for monoculture cultivation may lead to water scarcity in certain regions. Conservation-oriented approaches advocate for water-efficient cultivation methods like rain-fed agriculture and water recycling systems. These practices minimize the environmental impact and enhance the resilience of herb cultivation in the face of climate variability.

Fair wild harvesting is a fundamental component of conservation initiatives in areas where wildcrafted herbs constitute a substantial economic resource for nearby communities. Overuse of wild plant populations can result in social unrest, economic inequality, and the loss of traditional knowledge. Demands from outside markets frequently cause this overuse. Conservation efforts aim to alleviate these problems by encouraging fair trade methods and ensuring that local communities are fairly compensated for their contributions to the herbal sector. Involving local stakeholders in decision-making processes, collaborative projects support community-led conservation activities consistent with social and environmental sustainability.

Certification programs and standards, such as the FairWild Standard, provide frameworks for conservation-oriented practices in wild harvesting. These certifications aim to ensure that the collection of wild plants is sustainable, socially responsible, and environmentally conscious. Adhering to established standards, herbal companies demonstrate their commitment to conservation efforts and responsible sourcing. By purchasing goods that have official certifications, consumers can make educated decisions and encourage the herbal sector to adopt more conservation-focused methods.

Another problem influencing conservation efforts in the herbal sector is climate change. Identifying plant species resilient to climate change, promoting agroecological practices that increase ecosystem resilience, and developing adaptable techniques for growing herbs are among conservation initiatives in response to this phenomenon. The herbal industry, environmental organizations, and academic institutions must work together to address the complex and dynamic issues posed by climate change.

Education campaigns are essential to conservation efforts because they raise people's knowledge and comprehension of how herbal practices affect the environment. Through promoting sustainable harvesting, production, and consumption methods, education enables individuals, practitioners, and corporations to make educated decisions consistent with conservation aims. Including environmental education in public outreach initiatives and herbal training programs helps foster a shared commitment to ethical and ecological herbal activities.

In conclusion, the environmental impact of herbal medicine is a multifaceted issue that requires concerted conservation efforts. Sustainable harvesting, cultivation practices, biodiversity conservation, fair trade, water resource management, climate resilience, and educational initiatives collectively contribute to a holistic approach to environmental sustainability within the herbal industry. As the demand for herbal products rises, integrating conservation-oriented practices becomes increasingly urgent. The herbal business may significantly protect the planet's biodiversity, assist local people, and foster a more sustainable and healthful future by adopting responsible environmental stewardship.

Ethical considerations in herbal medicine production

Ethical considerations in herbal medicine production within Chinese medicine are of paramount importance, reflecting a commitment to values that extend beyond profit margins to encompass sustainability, cultural integrity, and social responsibility. Traditional Chinese medicine (TCM), with its rich history and reliance on diverse plant species, is deeply entwined with ethical considerations that shape the entire production process—from cultivation and harvesting to processing and distribution.

One primary ethical concern in herbal medicine production is sourcing and harvesting medicinal plants. Overharvesting, driven by increasing global demand, threatens the sustainability of certain plant species, particularly those with specific therapeutic properties. Responsible sourcing practices emphasize ethical wildcrafting and sustainable cultivation methods, ensuring that the collection of herbs aligns with ecological principles and allows for the regeneration of plant populations. By prioritizing the well-being of plant ecosystems, ethical considerations in sourcing safeguard the integrity of herbal medicine and contribute to the conservation of biodiversity.

Cultivation practices, another critical facet of herbal medicine production, raise ethical considerations regarding environmental sustainability and land use. Large-scale monoculture, accompanied by the extensive use of synthetic fertilizers and pesticides, can result in soil degradation, loss of biodiversity, and negative impacts on surrounding ecosystems. Ethical approaches to cultivation advocate for agroecological methods that prioritize soil health, promote biodiversity and minimize environmental harm. Organic farming practices, which eschew synthetic inputs in favor of natural and sustainable alternatives, align with ethical considerations that seek to harmonize herbal cultivation with ecological well-being.

Fair labor practices are integral to the ethical considerations in herbal medicine production, particularly in regions where traditional herbs are grown, harvested, and processed. Ensuring that the individuals involved in herb cultivation and harvesting are treated ethically, receive fair compensation, and work in safe conditions is essential for fostering a socially responsible herbal industry. Ethical sourcing initiatives emphasize transparency in the supply chain, traceability of herbs from cultivation to distribution, and adherence to fair labor standards. By prioritizing the well-being of those engaged in the herbal trade, ethical considerations contribute to creating a more equitable and socially conscious herbal industry.

One of the central tenets of ethical concerns in manufacturing Chinese herbal medicine is maintaining cultural integrity. Chinese culture has long been the foundation of traditional Chinese medicine, and regional customs and traditions are closely linked to numerous drugs. Collaborating with local communities, honoring indigenous knowledge, and appreciating the cultural relevance of herbal practices are all components of ethical production processes. As local practitioners and communities take on the role of stewards of their herbal traditions, this strategy guarantees the preservation of priceless cultural heritage. It promotes a sense of empowerment within the community.

Quality control and safety are fundamental ethical considerations in herbal medicine production. Ensuring herbal products' purity, authenticity, and safety is crucial for consumer trust and well-being. Ethical producers prioritize rigorous testing for contaminants, accurate identification of plant species, and adherence to quality standards. By maintaining a commitment to product integrity, ethical considerations underscore the responsibility of herbal producers to provide safe and effective remedies to consumers.

The concept of sustainability extends beyond ecological considerations to encompass economic sustainability and social equity. Ethical considerations in herbal medicine production emphasize the importance of fair trade practices that ensure local communities receive fair compensation for their contributions to the herbal industry. Collaborative initiatives involve local stakeholders in decision-making processes, fostering community-led conservation efforts that align with environmental and social sustainability. Ethical producers recognize the interconnectedness of economic and ecological well-being, striving to create a herbal industry that benefits local communities and the planet.

Certification programs and standards, such as Good Manufacturing Practices (GMP) and organic certifications, offer frameworks for ethical herbal medicine production. These certifications guide responsible sourcing, cultivation practices, and quality control measures. By adhering to established standards, ethical producers demonstrate their commitment to ethical considerations and contribute to the overall sustainability and credibility of the herbal industry.

In the age of globalization, ethical considerations also extend to fair and respectful engagement with traditional knowledge. Indigenous and local communities often hold valuable knowledge about the uses and cultivation of medicinal plants. Ethical herbal medicine production involves collaborative partnerships that recognize, respect, and compensate these communities for their traditional knowledge. By fostering equitable relationships, ethical producers contribute to preserving conventional wisdom and acknowledging the cultural heritage embedded in herbal medicine.

Educational initiatives are crucial components of ethical considerations in herbal medicine production. By raising awareness about sustainable practices, fair trade, and the cultural importance of herbal traditions, education empowers individuals, practitioners, and businesses to make informed and ethical choices. Integrating ethical considerations into herbal training programs, public outreach campaigns, and consumer education contributes to a shared commitment to responsible and sustainable herbal practices.

In summary, ethical issues surrounding the manufacture of herbal medicines in Chinese medicine represent a comprehensive dedication to social responsibility, cultural integrity, and sustainability. The herbal business can positively impact a more responsible and ethical future by adopting ethical sourcing, cultivation procedures, fair labor standards, and quality control systems. Integrating these factors into the manufacturing of herbal medicines becomes both a moral requirement and a calculated decision for creating a robust and well-respected herbal sector, as customers seek out products more closely linked with ethical principles.

CHAPTER X
Challenges and Misconceptions

Addressing common misconceptions about Chinese herbal medicine

Addressing common misconceptions about Chinese herbal medicine is crucial for fostering a comprehensive understanding of this ancient healing tradition, dispelling myths, and encouraging informed choices among individuals seeking alternative and complementary approaches to healthcare. One prevalent misconception is the belief that Chinese herbal medicine is solely based on superstition or folklore rather than grounded in systematic and empirical observations. Chinese herbal medicine has developed over millennia, guided by extensive clinical experience, recorded in classical literature, and furthered by current research and contemporary uses.

Safety concerns are another common misperception; some people believe that using Chinese herbal medicine carries hazards or adverse consequences. Chinese herbal medicine has a long usage history, and careful attention to herbal formulations emphasizes their safety. It is true that any kind of therapy, including herbal medicines, should be used cautiously and under the advice of qualified practitioners. To reduce the possibility of adverse reactions, Traditional Chinese Medicine (TCM) strongly emphasizes customized prescriptions, in which herbal formulae are meticulously matched to each patient's unique constitutional needs and medical conditions.

Another widespread misconception is that Chinese herbal medicine functions independently of conventional medicine, leading to an untrue binary opposition. An integrative strategy that draws on the advantages of conventional and traditional medicine is frequently recommended. Combining Chinese herbal medicine with conventional therapies has several advantages, especially when dealing with complicated or persistent medical conditions. Realizing the complementarity and compatibility of these approaches paves the way for a more thorough and patient-centered approach to healthcare.

The complexity of Chinese herbal medicine formulations often leads to the misconception that they are challenging to understand or administer without specialized knowledge. While it is true that herbal medicine requires expertise for optimal results, this should not discourage individuals from exploring its potential benefits. Qualified Chinese medicine practitioners undergo extensive training, learning to assess individual health conditions, diagnose underlying imbalances, and formulate customized herbal prescriptions. Seeking guidance from a skilled practitioner ensures that the complexities of Chinese herbal medicine are navigated effectively, providing personalized and targeted support.

Some individuals may also mistakenly believe that Chinese herbal medicine is exclusively rooted in ancient principles and has yet to evolve to integrate modern scientific insights. In reality, ongoing research in China and the global scientific community continually validates and refines the understanding of Chinese herbal medicine. Numerous studies explore the pharmacological properties, mechanisms of action, and clinical efficacy of individual herbs and herbal formulations. Integrating traditional wisdom with contemporary scientific findings allows for a more comprehensive and evidence-based approach to herbal medicine.

The notion that Chinese herbal medicine is a one-size-fits-all solution is a common oversimplification. In contrast, TCM principles emphasize the importance of individualized treatment plans. Each person's constitution, health history, and presenting symptoms are carefully considered in the formulation of herbal prescriptions. Rather than only providing short-term symptom alleviation, this customized strategy targets the underlying causes of health problems, encouraging long- term balance and well-being.

Another misconception involves the belief that Chinese herbal medicine is exclusively plant-based. While plants constitute a significant portion of herbal remedies, Chinese medicine also incorporates minerals and animal products. Substances such as pearls, shells, and certain animal-derived ingredients are used judiciously based on their therapeutic properties and historical applications. Understanding the diverse range of substances employed in Chinese herbal medicine provides a more accurate appreciation of its holistic and inclusive approach to healing.

Some individuals may hesitate to explore Chinese herbal medicine due to concerns about its taste or form of administration. The perception that herbal formulas are unpalatable or difficult to incorporate into daily routines is a misconception that overlooks the adaptability of these remedies. Modern formulations often come in various convenient forms, including capsules, pills, granules, or liquid extracts. Moreover, the taste of herbal teas can be adjusted, and practitioners work collaboratively with individuals to find formulations that are effective, palatable, and easy to incorporate into daily life.

There is also a common misconception that Chinese herbal medicine is a last resort, sought only when conventional treatments have failed. In reality, many individuals turn to Chinese herbal medicine as a proactive and preventative healthcare strategy or complementary approach to enhance overall well-being. The holistic nature of Chinese medicine allows for addressing specific symptoms and underlying imbalances and promoting preventive measures to maintain optimal health.

Lastly, the notion that Chinese herbal medicine needs more scientific validation is a misconception that must be addressed in the substantial body of research supporting its efficacy. Numerous studies have explored Chinese herbal medicine's pharmacological actions, safety profiles, and clinical outcomes. In addition, the World Health Organization (WHO) and various national health agencies recognize the value of traditional medicine, including Chinese herbal medicine, in healthcare systems. Integrating this wealth of scientific evidence with conventional knowledge contributes to a more nuanced and evidence-based understanding of Chinese herbal medicine.

In conclusion, addressing common misconceptions about Chinese herbal medicine is essential for fostering informed perspectives and encouraging individuals to explore the potential benefits of this ancient healing tradition. By dispelling myths related to safety, compatibility with conventional medicine, complexity, and taste, individuals can approach Chinese herbal medicine with a more accurate understanding of its principles, practices, and modern applications. The collaboration between traditional wisdom and scientific insights continues to shape Chinese herbal medicine as a dynamic and evolving healthcare system, offering valuable contributions to holistic well-being.

Overcoming skepticism and cultural barriers

Overcoming skepticism and cultural barriers regarding Chinese medicines is a multifaceted endeavor that involves addressing misconceptions, fostering cross-cultural understanding, and highlighting the integrative potential of traditional Chinese medicine (TCM) within diverse healthcare landscapes. Skepticism often arises due to differences in cultural perspectives, varying medical paradigms, and a need for more familiarity with Chinese medicine principles. To bridge these gaps and encourage a more open-minded approach, it is essential to explore Chinese medicines' historical context, philosophical foundations, and clinical efficacy.

Historically, Chinese medicine has evolved over thousands of years, making it one of the world's oldest continuously practiced medical systems. Its enduring legacy attests to its cultural significance and the effectiveness of its approaches. Skepticism can be addressed by recognizing the wealth of empirical knowledge that underlies Chinese medicine, with its roots in careful observation, clinical experience, and the systematic recording of therapeutic practices over generations. Understanding the historical development of Chinese medicine provides a context that challenges the perception of it being merely a collection of outdated or superstitious beliefs.

These concepts may seem unfamiliar or abstract to those more accustomed to Western medical paradigms, leading to skepticism about the validity of Chinese medical theories. However, a deeper exploration of these principles reveals a sophisticated understanding of the body as a dynamic and interconnected system. By recognizing the subtle interplay of Yin and Yang forces and the importance of maintaining equilibrium for optimal health, individuals can appreciate Chinese medicine's holistic and preventive aspects.

The clinical efficacy of Chinese medicines is a critical aspect of overcoming skepticism. While traditional approaches may differ from Western diagnostic methods and treatments, numerous studies have demonstrated the effectiveness of Chinese herbal medicine, acupuncture, and other modalities in addressing various health conditions. Research exploring the pharmacological actions, mechanisms of action, and clinical outcomes associated with Chinese medicines contributes to a growing body of evidence that supports their therapeutic potential. Highlighting the scientific validation of Chinese medicines helps build credibility and fosters confidence among skeptics.

Cultural obstacles are frequently the result of a need for knowledge or comprehension of Chinese medical concepts and procedures. To overcome this, educational programs are critical in promoting intercultural understanding and demystifying Chinese medicine. Myths can be debunked, misconceptions can be cleared up, and a more open-minded and knowledgeable viewpoint can be enabled by incorporating Chinese medicine into mainstream healthcare education and public awareness initiatives. Education should emphasize the comprehensive nature of Chinese medicine and its integration of mind, body, and spirit, going beyond the clinical elements and delving into the cultural background.

Language can be a significant barrier when communicating about Chinese medicines. Technical terms, cultural nuances, and the unique language of Chinese medical theories may pose challenges for individuals unfamiliar with the terminology. Translating these concepts into accessible language and providing clear explanations can enhance understanding and bridge linguistic gaps. Moreover, fostering open and respectful dialogue between practitioners of different medical traditions facilitates mutual learning and dispels preconceived notions, promoting a collaborative approach to healthcare.

In the context of overcoming skepticism, acknowledging the limitations of any medical system is crucial. Chinese medicine is not a panacea, and its efficacy can vary based on individual responses and the nature of health conditions. An honest and transparent discussion about the strengths and limitations of Chinese medicines contributes to building trust and credibility. Practitioners and educators should emphasize the importance of an integrative approach to healthcare, recognizing that different medical traditions can complement each other for the patient's benefit.

Cultural competence in healthcare is essential for overcoming barriers related to cultural differences. Understanding diverse cultural perspectives, beliefs, and practices contributes to more effective communication and fosters trust between healthcare providers and patients. To guarantee courteous and patient-centered care, cultural competence training for medical practitioners should cover knowledge of traditional therapeutic modalities, such as those found in Chinese medicine. Healthcare professionals who recognize and consider different cultural viewpoints can foster a more welcoming and inclusive atmosphere.

One effective strategy for overcoming skepticism is integrating Chinese medicine into mainstream healthcare systems. Collaborative efforts between Western and traditional Chinese medicine allow for a more comprehensive and patient-centered approach. Integrative healthcare models, where practitioners from different traditions work collaboratively to address patients' needs, have gained traction in various parts of the world. Such models recognize the strengths of each system and leverage their complementary nature to provide more comprehensive and personalized care.

Community engagement and grassroots initiatives also play a crucial role in overcoming skepticism and cultural barriers. By involving local communities and providing platforms for dialogue, individuals can share their experiences with Chinese medicine, dispel myths, and offer insights into its cultural significance. Community-based educational programs, workshops, and events create spaces for individuals to ask questions, voice concerns, and gain firsthand knowledge about Chinese medicines. Engaging communities empowers individuals to make informed choices about their healthcare and encourages a more open-minded approach to diverse healing traditions.

Research and evidence-based practice are pivotal in overcoming skepticism regarding Chinese medicines. Continued research into the mechanisms of action, safety profiles, and clinical efficacy of Chinese herbal medicine, acupuncture, and other modalities strengthens the evidence base supporting these practices. Collaboration between researchers from different medical traditions contributes to a more comprehensive understanding of healthcare practices, fostering a shared commitment to evidence-based care. Integrating Chinese medicine into research and academic settings helps legitimize its place within the broader healthcare landscape.

In conclusion, overcoming skepticism and cultural barriers regarding Chinese medicines requires a multifaceted approach that addresses historical, philosophical, and clinical aspects while fostering cross-cultural understanding. Education, research, integrative healthcare models, community engagement, and cultural competence training are essential to this transformative process. By recognizing the strengths and limitations of different medical traditions, fostering open dialogue, and promoting collaborative approaches to healthcare, individuals and healthcare systems can embrace the diversity of healing traditions to benefit global well-being.

Navigating challenges in integrating traditional practices with modern healthcare

Navigating challenges in integrating traditional practices with modern healthcare is a complex endeavor that involves reconciling diverse perspectives, addressing regulatory considerations, fostering cross-disciplinary collaboration, and promoting patient-centered care. Integrating traditional practices, such as traditional Chinese medicine (TCM), Ayurveda, or herbal remedies, with modern healthcare reflects a recognition of the valuable contributions of diverse healing traditions. However, this integration has challenges, as it requires navigating cultural, philosophical, and methodological differences while ensuring patient safety, evidence-based practice, and regulatory compliance.

Cultural and philosophical differences between traditional and modern healthcare systems can present significant challenges in the integration process. Traditional healing practices often operate within holistic frameworks that consider the interconnectedness of the body, mind, and spirit. In contrast, modern medicine may lean towards reductionist approaches, focusing on specific symptoms and biochemical pathways. Bridging these philosophical gaps requires a mutual understanding and appreciation of the underlying principles of each system. Culturally competent healthcare providers can play a pivotal role in facilitating this dialogue, recognizing the strengths of traditional and modern approaches, and ensuring that patients receive care that respects their cultural preferences and beliefs.

Regulatory considerations pose another set of challenges in integrating traditional practices with modern healthcare. Traditional healing modalities often fall outside the regulatory frameworks established for conventional medicine. This lack of standardization can lead to concerns about safety, quality control, and consistency of care. Establishing clear regulatory guidelines that ensure the safety and efficacy of traditional practices without stifling their cultural richness is a delicate balance. Regulatory bodies need to collaborate with conventional practitioners, researchers, and policymakers to develop inclusive frameworks that recognize and legitimize the contributions of traditional healing systems within the broader healthcare landscape.

Integrating traditional practices also necessitates addressing the evidence-based practice paradigm prevalent in modern healthcare. Traditional healing systems often rely on empirical knowledge, experiential wisdom, and holistic approaches that may not align with the rigorous scientific methodologies commonly applied in modern medicine. To overcome this challenge, there is a growing need for research investigating the mechanisms of action, safety profiles, and clinical outcomes of traditional practices. Collaborative research initiatives between conventional healers, researchers, and healthcare institutions contribute to building an evidence base that supports the integration of effective conventional therapies into modern healthcare.

Interdisciplinary collaboration is a cornerstone of successful integration efforts, yet it brings its own set of challenges. Traditional practitioners and modern healthcare professionals may have different training, languages, and diagnostic approaches. Establishing effective communication channels and fostering mutual respect are essential for meaningful collaboration. These gaps are filled by interdisciplinary training programs, workshops, and shared learning experiences, which enable professionals from various backgrounds to comprehend one another's viewpoints and advance a more all-encompassing patient care strategy.

Patient-centered care, a fundamental principle in modern healthcare, becomes even more critical in integrating traditional practices. Patients often seek a blend of traditional and contemporary approaches to address their health concerns, emphasizing the importance of individualized and culturally sensitive care. Integrative healthcare models prioritizing patient preferences involve shared decision-making and offer therapeutic options that empower individuals to participate actively in their healing journey. Developing a solid patient-practitioner relationship built on trust and open communication is central to navigating the complexities of integrating traditional practices with modern healthcare.

Education plays a pivotal role in overcoming challenges associated with integration. Healthcare providers, students, and the public need access to accurate and unbiased information about traditional healing practices. Integrating education about traditional systems into medical and healthcare training programs helps foster a more inclusive understanding among future healthcare professionals. Public awareness campaigns can also be crucial in dispelling myths, addressing misconceptions, and promoting informed choices about integrating traditional practices with modern healthcare.

Cultural humility and respect for diverse worldviews are essential components of navigating challenges in integration. Acknowledging that traditional practices may have unique perspectives on health and illness fosters an environment where different healing traditions can coexist harmoniously. This cultural humility involves recognizing the historical context, acknowledging power differentials, and appreciating the richness of cultural diversity in healthcare. Training programs emphasizing cultural competence, empathy, and the importance of patient narratives contribute to creating a healthcare workforce better equipped to navigate the complexities of integrating traditional practices with modern healthcare.

Integrating traditional techniques requires careful attention to ethical issues, especially when honoring patient autonomy, informed consent, and preferences. Communicating openly and honestly about the advantages, drawbacks, and options for both conventional and contemporary approaches is crucial. Establishing trust in integrative healthcare environments requires adhering to ethical norms that prioritize patient well-being, respect cultural values, and secure anonymity. Collaboration and continuous communication between practitioners, ethicists, and politicians must balance the ethical principles of beneficence, autonomy, fairness, and non-maleficence.

The socio-economic context also plays a significant role in integrating traditional practices with modern healthcare. Economic factors, geographical location, and healthcare infrastructure may influence access to traditional healing modalities. Ensuring equitable access to conventional and contemporary healthcare options is crucial for promoting health justice. Integrative healthcare models prioritizing inclusivity and addressing disparities in access contribute to a more equitable healthcare system that recognizes and values diverse healing traditions.

Public perception and societal attitudes towards traditional practices can influence the success of integration efforts. Overcoming cultural biases, dispelling myths, and addressing stigmas associated with traditional healing is essential for fostering acceptance within the broader community. Advocacy campaigns, media representation, and community engagement initiatives shape positive attitudes toward integrating conventional practices with modern healthcare. Recognizing the cultural diversity within society and respecting individual choices in healthcare are essential components of fostering a supportive environment for integrative approaches.

In conclusion, navigating challenges in integrating traditional practices with modern healthcare requires a comprehensive and collaborative approach that addresses cultural, regulatory, educational, and ethical considerations. By fostering cross-disciplinary collaboration, promoting evidence-based practice, prioritizing patient-centered care, and addressing societal attitudes, healthcare systems can successfully integrate traditional healing practices to benefit diverse patient populations. Recognizing the value of conventional and modern approaches contributes to a more inclusive, holistic, and effective healthcare system that honors the cultural richness of healing traditions worldwide.

CHAPTER XI
Future Perspectives and Innovations

Evolving trends in Chinese Herbal Medicine

Evolving trends in Chinese Herbal Medicine reflect a dynamic interplay between traditional wisdom, modern research, and the changing landscape of healthcare preferences. Chinese Herbal Medicine (CHM) is an essential part of Traditional Chinese Medicine (TCM) and has a long history that dates back thousands of years. However, modern advances in science, technology, and medical care delivery have resulted in significant changes to how Chinese herbs are viewed, recommended, and incorporated into people's daily wellness routines worldwide.

One of the prominent trends in Chinese herbal medicine is the increasing recognition and acceptance of herbal medicine within mainstream healthcare systems. Historically, TCM and CHM were viewed skeptically outside traditional Chinese cultural contexts. However, as scientific research continues to explore Chinese herbs' pharmacological properties and clinical efficacy, these practices are gaining acknowledgment and integration into conventional healthcare settings. Healthcare professionals and institutions are exploring collaborative models that leverage the strengths of both traditional and modern medicine, providing patients with a more comprehensive and holistic approach to healthcare.

Personalized medicine has become a prominent trend in the larger healthcare field, and Chinese herbal therapy is not exempt from its influence. The significance of customized treatment based on each patient's distinct constitution, patterns of disharmony, and environmental factors has traditionally been emphasized in traditional

Chinese medicine. Recent technological developments, such as metabolomics and genetic testing, have made it possible to more precisely analyze individual differences in medication metabolism and reaction. This personalized approach aligns with the principles of TCM, allowing practitioners to tailor Chinese herbal formulations to each patient's specific needs and characteristics.

As consumer awareness and interest in holistic and preventative healthcare continue to rise, there is a growing trend towards using Chinese herbs for overall well-being rather than solely for addressing specific ailments. Individuals seek herbal formulations that support vitality, enhance resilience, and promote longevity. This shift reflects a broader cultural movement towards proactive health management and a recognition of the interconnectedness between physical, mental, and emotional well-being. Chinese herbal medicine, which emphasizes balance and harmony, aligns well with this preventive healthcare approach.

Another notable trend is the integration of Chinese Herbal Medicine into lifestyle practices, wellness routines, and complementary therapies. Traditional Chinese Medicine views health as a dynamic balance influenced by various factors, including diet, exercise, sleep, and emotional well-being. Integrating Chinese herbs into daily routines, such as herbal teas, dietary supplements, or topical applications, allows individuals to incorporate TCM principles into their lifestyle. This trend facilitates a more holistic approach to health and encourages a deeper connection with the natural world and the seasonal rhythms that influence well-being.

Collaboration and cross-disciplinary partnerships between Chinese medicine practitioners and professionals from other healthcare modalities represent a transformative trend in the field. Integrative healthcare models bring together the expertise of practitioners from different traditions, fostering a collaborative approach that addresses the complex needs of patients. Chinese Herbal Medicine is often integrated with acupuncture, nutritional therapy, mind-body practices, and conventional medicine to provide a comprehensive and patient-centered approach. This trend reflects a recognition of the value of diverse healing traditions working synergistically to benefit individual health.

As ecological responsibility has gained more attention globally, environmental sustainability has grown in importance when manufacturing and sourcing Chinese herbs. Overharvesting, habitat degradation, and unethical wildcrafting methods may threaten the availability and sustainability of some herbs. In response, a rising movement supports sustainable harvesting methods, nurturing endangered species, and engaging in ethical wildcrafting. Programs for certification, like the FairWild Standard, are designed to make sure that gathering wild plants is ethically and sustainably done, supporting fair trade principles and the welfare of nearby communities.

Innovation in herbal formulations and delivery methods is shaping the future of Chinese Herbal Medicine. Traditional methods of preparing herbal decoctions or teas complement modern formulations such as herbal extracts, granules, capsules, and topical applications. These innovations enhance convenience, dosage precision, and palatability, making Chinese herbal products more accessible and appealing to a broader audience. Additionally, research into novel delivery systems, such as nanotechnology and encapsulation, can improve Chinese herbs' bioavailability and therapeutic effects.

Digital technologies are revolutionizing the accessibility and distribution of knowledge on Chinese herbal medicine. Online platforms, mobile applications, and telehealth services can facilitate Chinese herbal product sales, consultations, and education. These technologies let people acquire trustworthy information on herbs and formulations, make remote consultations with Chinese medicine practitioners easier, and support the internationalization of Chinese herbal medicine. Integrating digital technologies does, however, bring up ethical issues, such as data security, privacy, and appropriate online information sharing.

Research into Chinese herbs' scientific mechanisms of action and pharmacological properties is expanding the evidence base supporting their use. While traditional knowledge and empirical observations have been the foundation of Chinese Herbal Medicine, modern research methodologies, including clinical trials, laboratory studies, and systematic reviews, contribute to a more nuanced understanding of Chinese herbs' therapeutic effects and safety profiles. This tendency promotes Chinese herbal medicine's legitimacy in the eyes of the larger medical community and helps patients and practitioners make well-informed decisions.

Chinese herbal medicine education and training are changing to satisfy the requirements of the public and healthcare professionals. More knowledgeable and culturally competent healthcare staff can be achieved by incorporating Chinese medicine principles into traditional healthcare education, providing self-directed learning tools, and continuing education programs. Incorporating Chinese Herbal Medicine into recognized educational establishments and joint ventures with conventional medical schools signifies a broader recognition of the significance of classic therapeutic methods in contemporary healthcare.

Cultivating partnerships between China and other countries is influencing the globalization of Chinese Herbal Medicine. Collaborative research initiatives, international conferences, and exchanging knowledge and expertise contribute to a more interconnected global community of Chinese medicine practitioners. This trend facilitates cross-cultural dialogue, enables the sharing of best practices, and supports the integration of Chinese Herbal Medicine into diverse healthcare systems worldwide. However, it also raises challenges related to standardization, cultural adaptation, and the need for respectful engagement with various healing traditions.

In conclusion, evolving trends in Chinese Herbal Medicine reflect a dynamic intersection of tradition, innovation, and global influences. The integration of Chinese Herbal Medicine into mainstream healthcare, personalized approaches, preventive healthcare strategies, lifestyle integration, collaboration with other healthcare modalities, environmental sustainability, innovation in formulations, digital technologies, scientific research, education, and global partnerships collectively contribute to the ongoing evolution of this ancient healing tradition. As Chinese Herbal Medicine continues to adapt to the changing landscape of healthcare, it offers a valuable and holistic approach to promoting well-being and addressing the complex health challenges of the modern world.

Integration with modern medicine and scientific research

Integrating Chinese Herbal Medicine (CHM) with modern medicine and scientific research represents a transformative and dynamic convergence of traditional wisdom and contemporary evidence-based practices. Traditional Chinese Medicine (TCM), of which CHM is integral, has a rich history dating back thousands of years, rooted in ancient philosophies and empirical observations. In recent decades, there has been a significant shift towards integrating CHM into mainstream healthcare systems, fostering collaboration between traditional practitioners and modern medical professionals.

Scientific investigation has primarily confirmed Chinese herbal mixtures' safety and medicinal efficacy. The foundation of Chinese herbal medicine (CHM) is traditional knowledge. Still, thorough scientific studies have given us a more complete understanding of different plants' pharmacological characteristics, modes of action, and therapeutic uses. Several investigations have examined the molecular components of Chinese herbs, pinpointed their bioactive contents, and clarified their influence on physiological mechanisms. This scientific examination helps to establish an evidence base that supports the historical application of CHM and directs its incorporation into contemporary healthcare.

The frequency of clinical trials assessing Chinese herbal formulations' efficacy has increased, bringing CHM into line with the methodological standards demanded by contemporary medical research. For various medical problems, randomized controlled trials, systematic reviews, and meta-analyses offer insightful information about the therapeutic results of CHM therapies. Scientific research has been conducted on diseases like gynecological illnesses, respiratory disorders, gastrointestinal problems, and chronic pain. This research has provided information on the safety and effectiveness of many herbal remedies. The increasing data from these studies helps patients and practitioners make well-informed decisions.

Beyond research, CHM is incorporated into collaborative patient care approaches in modern medicine. Acknowledging the potential advantages of an integrative approach, some healthcare facilities have set up departments or clinics providing both traditional and mainstream therapies. Patients can receive CHM in addition to conventional treatment thanks to integrative medicine, which blends the best aspects of many healing techniques. Collaborative care models promote a more thorough and patient-centered approach to treatment by facilitating communication and coordination between traditional Chinese medicine practitioners and allopathic physicians.

Personalized medicine, a burgeoning paradigm in modern healthcare, resonates closely with the principles of CHM. Traditional Chinese Medicine has long emphasized the importance of individualized treatment based on a person's constitution, patterns of disharmony, and environmental influences. With advancements in genetics, metabolomics, and other fields, personalized medicine is gaining prominence in traditional and modern healthcare. Genetic variations, lifestyle factors, and individual responses to treatment are considered in tailoring CHM prescriptions, aligning the practice with the precision medicine approach that is increasingly valued in modern medical care.

One significant way Chinese herbal medicines have been incorporated into contemporary healthcare is as adjuvants to conventional treatments. CHM is frequently used with pharmaceutical therapies to improve therapeutic outcomes and reduce adverse effects. This cooperative approach is especially noticeable in cancer patients, as CHM formulations enhance immune function, reduce symptoms, and enhance general health in patients receiving traditional treatments. The integration of CHM into cancer care reflects a complete strategy that considers the psychological and physical aspects of the patient's experience.

The perspective of Traditional Chinese Medicine emphasizes the connection between the mind and body, viewing mental and emotional health as essential to general health. Studies examining the neuropharmacological impacts of specific Chinese herbs, especially those possessing adaptogenic qualities, exhibit the potential to manage ailments such as stress, anxiety, and depression. Integrating CHM with psychotherapy and psychotropic drugs is a reflection of a comprehensive approach to mental health that recognizes the complex interplay between psychological health and well-being.

While integration with modern medicine offers numerous opportunities, it also poses challenges related to standardization, quality control, and communication between practitioners of different modalities. Standardizing herbal formulations, ensuring product consistency, and addressing contamination issues are crucial considerations in the safe integration of CHM into modern healthcare. Regulatory frameworks play a significant role in overseeing the quality and safety of herbal products, necessitating collaboration between traditional medicine regulators and conventional healthcare authorities.

Scientific research has also explored the safety profiles and potential herb-drug interactions associated with Chinese herbal medicines. Understanding herbal compounds' pharmacokinetics and pharmacodynamics helps practitioners make informed decisions about combining CHM with pharmaceutical drugs. Preventing negative interactions and improving patient outcomes in integrated care settings need open communication between patients and healthcare professionals and cooperation between practitioners of traditional Chinese medicine and allopathic physicians.

Education and training represent critical components of the successful integration of CHM into modern healthcare. Traditional Chinese medicine practitioners seeking collaboration with allopathic physicians benefit from understanding Western medical diagnostics, terminology, and treatment protocols. Similarly, modern healthcare professionals engaging with CHM need knowledge about traditional diagnostic methods, herbal formulations, and the holistic principles of Traditional Chinese Medicine. Cross-disciplinary educational initiatives, joint training programs, and ongoing professional development contribute to creating a healthcare workforce well-versed in traditional and modern approaches.

Patient awareness and acceptance of CHM within modern healthcare are also significant factors in the integration process. Public education campaigns, information dissemination, and collaborative efforts between traditional and contemporary healthcare practitioners contribute to a more informed patient population. Giving people the information, they need to make decisions about their healthcare, such as whether to include CHM in their treatment plans, increases patient autonomy and promotes a sense of collaboration in the healing process.

The internationalization of CHM is a notable trend, with Chinese herbal medicines gaining popularity beyond traditional cultural contexts. As research highlights the therapeutic potential of specific herbs, formulations, and acupuncture techniques, interest in CHM has spread globally. This trend is reflected in the establishment of TCM clinics and educational institutions outside of China and the incorporation of CHM into integrative medicine practices in diverse healthcare settings. Cross-cultural collaborations contribute to mutually enriching traditional healing practices and modern medical knowledge.

In conclusion, integrating Chinese Herbal Medicine with modern medicine and scientific research represents a transformative journey of collaboration, evidence-based practices, and a holistic approach to patient care. The alignment of CHM with personalized medicine, the use of herbal adjuvants in conventional treatments, the integration into mental health care, and the challenges related to standardization and education collectively shape the evolving landscape of this ancient healing tradition. As the integration of CHM into modern healthcare continues to advance, it offers a unique and valuable contribution to the diverse tapestry of therapeutic options available to individuals seeking comprehensive and personalized healthcare solutions.

The potential for continued growth and development

Chinese Herbal Medicine (CHM) has enormous potential for future growth and development due to various factors, including growing interest in holistic healthcare worldwide and ongoing scientific studies confirming the medicinal benefits of traditional Chinese herbs. The holistic and individualized approach CHM provides is becoming increasingly recognized as the world struggles with the complexity of modern healthcare, opening the door for broader integration of this method into standard medical practices.

One key driver of the potential growth of CHM lies in the increasing awareness and acceptance of holistic and preventative healthcare approaches. Traditional Chinese Medicine (TCM), of which CHM is integral, views health as a state of balance and harmony within the body. This holistic perspective aligns with a global shift towards recognizing the interconnectedness of physical, mental, and emotional well-being. As individuals seek comprehensive and patient-centered care, the principles of CHM resonate, offering a unique lens through which to address the root causes of health issues and promote overall well-being.

The rise of personalized medicine is another influential factor contributing to the growth of CHM. Traditional Chinese Medicine has long emphasized the importance of tailoring treatments to individual characteristics, including constitution, lifestyle, and patterns of disharmony. With advancements in genetic testing, metabolomics, and other personalized medicine technologies, there is a growing alignment between the principles of CHM and the modern approach to precision medicine. This convergence creates opportunities for CHM to play a pivotal role in providing individualized and targeted therapeutic interventions based on a person's unique health profile.

Scientific research continues to be a driving force behind the growth of CHM, offering insights into the mechanisms of action, safety profiles, and clinical applications of traditional Chinese herbs. The rigorous investigation of herbal formulations through randomized controlled trials, systematic reviews, and meta-analyses contributes to the evidence base supporting the use of CHM across a spectrum of health conditions. Integrating scientific knowledge with traditional wisdom enhances the credibility of CHM, fostering trust among healthcare professionals and the general public and positioning it as a valuable component of modern healthcare.

The growth potential also extends to the integration of CHM into mainstream healthcare systems globally. Collaborative models that combine traditional Chinese medicine practitioners and allopathic physicians are gaining traction, creating an environment where patients can access the benefits of conventional and modern medical approaches. As healthcare institutions establish integrative medicine departments and clinics, CHM becomes integral to a more comprehensive and patient- centered healthcare landscape. This trend signifies a departure from the historical compartmentalization of traditional and modern medicine, offering a holistic approach that leverages both strengths.

Environmental sustainability considerations are increasingly shaping CHM's growth trajectory. As awareness of ecological impact and conservation efforts grows, a heightened focus is on responsible sourcing, ethical wildcrafting, and sustainable cultivation practices for Chinese herbs. Certification programs such as the FairWild Standard, which promotes sustainable and socially accountable wild plant harvesting, contribute to ensuring the long-term availability of medicinal plants. This environmentally conscious approach aligns with broader global efforts towards ethical and sustainable healthcare practices, positioning CHM as a responsible and ecologically aware choice.

Innovation in herbal formulations and delivery methods is another avenue for the continued growth of CHM. Modern formulations such as herbal extracts, granules, capsules, and topical applications complement traditional methods of preparing decoctions. These innovations enhance convenience, dosage precision, and palatability, making Chinese herbal products more accessible and appealing to a broader audience. Research into novel delivery systems, such as nanotechnology and encapsulation, can improve Chinese herbs' bioavailability and therapeutic effects, further expanding their applications in healthcare.

International collaborations and partnerships facilitate the integration of CHM into global healthcare systems. As countries exchange knowledge, research findings, and best practices, CHM becomes a shared resource that transcends cultural boundaries. Collaborative efforts in research, education, and clinical practice contribute to the mutual enrichment of traditional healing practices and modern medical knowledge. This cross-cultural exchange fosters a global community of practitioners and researchers who are collectively advancing the understanding and utilization of CHM.

The potential growth of CHM is intricately tied to ongoing educational initiatives that bridge the gap between traditional and modern healthcare practices. Integrating Chinese medicine principles into mainstream healthcare education, offering cross-disciplinary training programs, and providing resources for self-directed learning contribute to a more informed and culturally competent healthcare workforce. The integration of CHM into accredited academic institutions and collaborative programs with conventional medical schools reflects a broader acknowledgment of the value of traditional healing practices in modern healthcare. Education empowers practitioners and raises awareness and acceptance among the general public, fostering a more informed and receptive attitude toward CHM.

In mental health, the potential for growth in the utilization of CHM is gaining prominence. Traditional Chinese Medicine views mental and emotional well-being as integral to overall health, emphasizing the interconnectedness of the mind and body. Scientific research exploring the neuropharmacological effects of certain Chinese herbs, such as those with adaptogenic properties, shows promise in addressing conditions like anxiety, depression, and stress. The integrative use of CHM with psychotherapy and psychotropic medications reflects a holistic approach to mental health that acknowledges the multifaceted nature of psychological well-being. As the demand for holistic mental health solutions grows, CHM stands poised to contribute significantly to this evolving field.

Digital technologies are serving as catalysts for the growth of CHM by enhancing accessibility, information dissemination, and consultation services. Online platforms, mobile applications, and telehealth services provide avenues for education, consultation, and purchasing Chinese herbal products. These technologies bridge geographical barriers, enabling individuals to consult with Chinese medicine practitioners remotely and access reliable information about herbs and formulations. The digitization of healthcare also facilitates research collaboration, data sharing, and the globalization of CHM knowledge, contributing to its continued growth on a global scale.

The potential for growth in CHM has its challenges. Standardization, quality control, and regulatory considerations are critical aspects that need continued attention to ensure the safety and efficacy of Chinese herbal products. Ethical considerations related to responsible sourcing, fair trade practices, and the preservation of cultural knowledge also play a crucial role in the sustainable development of CHM. Addressing these challenges requires ongoing collaboration between traditional medicine regulators, healthcare authorities, and the herbal industry to establish guidelines that promote ethical and environmentally conscious practices.

In conclusion, the potential for the continued growth and development of Chinese Herbal Medicine is anchored in a confluence of factors, including increasing global interest in holistic healthcare, ongoing scientific research, integration into mainstream healthcare, environmental sustainability efforts, innovation in formulations, international collaborations, educational initiatives, mental health applications, and the leveraging of digital technologies. As CHM continues to evolve and adapt to the changing landscape of healthcare, its unique contributions to holistic well-being position it as a valuable and dynamic component of the global healthcare system. The growth journey for CHM involves not only advancing its scientific understanding but also fostering a deeper appreciation for its cultural richness and potential to contribute to a more balanced, personalized, and sustainable approach to healthcare worldwide.

CHAPTER XII
Cultural and Spiritual Dimensions of Chinese Herbal Medicine

Chinese Medicine as a Lifestyle

Chinese Medicine transcends the conventional realm of healthcare; it embodies a holistic lifestyle that interweaves ancient wisdom with daily practices, promoting a harmonious balance between mind, body, and spirit. Embracing Chinese Medicine as a lifestyle involves seeking remedies for ailments and adopting a proactive approach to well-being that aligns with the principles of traditional Chinese philosophy. Central to this lifestyle is the concept of balance, inspired by the interplay of Yin and Yang forces. Incorporating elements of Chinese Medicine into daily routines fosters equilibrium, acknowledging the cyclical nature of life and the dynamic interdependence of opposites.

Chinese Medicine encourages individuals to be attuned to their bodies, recognizing the subtle signs of imbalance and taking preventive measures to restore harmony. Dietary habits play a pivotal role in this lifestyle, emphasizing consuming foods that correspond to the seasons and align with individual constitutions. The Five Elements theory, integral to Chinese Medicine, guides dietary choices, connecting the flavors of foods with specific organ systems and their corresponding elemental attributes.

Beyond dietary considerations, the lifestyle encompasses movement practices that harmonize Qi flow and cultivate physical strength. Tai Chi and Qi Gong, ancient Chinese exercises rooted in martial arts and meditation, are embraced as forms of physical activity and mindful practices that align the body's energies. These exercises contribute to flexibility, balance, and groundedness, promoting overall well-being.

Herbal teas, a staple in Chinese households, are integrated seamlessly into this lifestyle. Beyond their medicinal properties, these teas are cherished for their ability to connect individuals with the healing power of nature.

Cultivating mindfulness is another cornerstone of the Chinese Medicine lifestyle. The practice of mindful eating, where individuals savor each bite and appreciate the nourishment provided by the food, extends to broader mindfulness in daily activities. Mindful living involves being present at the moment, whether during a daily walk, a conversation, or preparing a meal. This awareness reduces stress, enhances mental clarity, and fosters a deeper connection with one's inner self.

The Chinese Medicine lifestyle encompasses the understanding that external factors, such as environmental changes and seasonal transitions, influence well-being. Individuals are encouraged to adapt their habits according to these shifts, aligning their activities with the rhythm of nature. This attunement to the seasons extends to clothing choices, sleep patterns, and overall daily routines, reflecting the acknowledgment of the interconnectedness between the internal and external worlds.

Furthermore, the lifestyle promotes emotional well-being by recognizing emotions' integral role in health. According to Chinese Medicine, emotions are interconnected with specific organ systems, and an imbalance in emotions can affect the corresponding organs. Acupuncture, herbal medicines, and mindfulness exercises are among the practices that strive to balance emotional states to promote emotional resilience and uphold mental equilibrium.

In essence, Chinese Medicine as a lifestyle is an invitation to live in harmony with the natural order, recognizing the interdependence of all things. It is a philosophy that transcends individual health and extends to the broader community and environmental context. Embracing this lifestyle is not merely a set of practices but a holistic way of being that encourages individuals to cultivate a deeper connection with themselves, others, and the world around them. As more people seek comprehensive approaches to well-being, the Chinese Medicine lifestyle stands as a beacon, offering a timeless path to balance, vitality, and a harmonious existence.

Rituals and Practices for Holistic Living

Rituals and practices within traditional Chinese medicine (TCM) extend beyond mere routines; they form the foundation of holistic living, enriching the mind, body, and spirit with ancient wisdom. Central to these rituals is the concept of balance, rooted in the Yin-Yang philosophy and the harmonious flow of Qi, the vital life force. Morning rituals, often revered as a cornerstone of holistic living in Chinese tradition, commence with practices that awaken the body's energy and cultivate balance. These rituals often include exercises like Tai Chi or Qi Gong, gentle movements that enhance physical flexibility and mental focus. In addition, attentive exercises like breathing exercises or meditation are incorporated into morning rituals to promote serenity and create a positive atmosphere for the day.

The transition from day to night brings forth evening rituals, crucial for winding down and preparing the body for restorative sleep. Herbal teas, specifically chosen for their calming properties, take center stage. Chamomile, lavender, or blends containing adaptogenic herbs like reishi and ashwagandha are embraced for their soothing effects on the nervous system and for the symbolic act of connecting with nature's healing bounty. The evening ritual extends beyond herbal infusions to include activities encouraging relaxation, such as gentle stretching or reading, promoting a transition from the day's demands to a more serene state.

The significance of mealtime rituals in Chinese holistic living cannot be overstated. Beyond the nutritional aspect, meals are regarded as opportunities for nourishing the body and fostering a connection with loved ones. Mindful eating, a practice deeply ingrained in Chinese culture, involves savoring each bite, appreciating the flavors and textures, and nourishing oneself. This practice not only enhances digestion but also instills a sense of gratitude for the sustenance provided by the earth.

The changing seasons are acknowledged through specific rituals that align with the principles of the Five Elements, a fundamental aspect of Chinese philosophy. Seasonal rituals involve adapting one's diet, movement practices, and self-care routines to harmonize with the energies prevalent in each season. For example, spring may involve detoxifying herbs and embracing exercises that support the liver, while winter rituals may emphasize nourishing, warming foods and gentle movements to keep the kidneys.

Sleep, recognized as a vital component of holistic living, is surrounded by rituals to ensure restful and rejuvenating rest. Creating a calming bedtime routine, including activities like reading, gentle stretching, or practicing gratitude, signals to the body that it is time to unwind. Herbal infusions with soothing properties, such as valerian or passionflower, become a gentle intro to a refreshing night's sleep.

Beyond daily rituals, Chinese holistic living extends to broader practices that encompass the spiritual and cultural dimensions. Traditional festivals and celebrations provide community connection and alignment with nature's cycles. The Lunar New Year, for instance, is marked by festive gatherings and practices that signify renewal and the ushering in of positive energies. Another essential component of holistic living is Feng Shui, the ancient Chinese art of balancing one's surroundings. It helps people design environments that promote harmony and well-being.

Deeply ingrained in Chinese medicine, acupuncture is both a curative and ritual to balance and harmonize Qi flow. Frequent acupuncture appointments become a sacred time for self-care, balancing the body's energies and treating imbalances before they appear as mental or physical symptoms.

In conclusion, rituals and practices for holistic living within the realm of traditional Chinese medicine transcend routine; they embody a philosophy that acknowledges the interconnectedness of the individual with nature, the community, and the cosmos. These rituals are not mere acts; they are intentional expressions of reverence for the body, gratitude for the sustenance provided by the earth, and a commitment to living in harmony with the rhythms of life. Through daily and seasonal rituals, Chinese holistic living becomes a way of being, an ongoing celebration of balance, vitality, and a holistic connection with the essence of existence. In embracing these practices, individuals embark on a journey that transcends the physical, nurturing a state of well-being that encompasses the mind, body, and spirit.

Connecting with Nature and the Seasons

Connecting with nature and the seasons is at the heart of traditional Chinese medicine (TCM), a profound philosophy recognizing the intimate relationship between human health and the natural world. In the tapestry of TCM, the changing seasons are not merely markers of weather transitions but reflections of the dynamic interplay of Yin and Yang energies. Each season is associated with specific elements, organ systems, and emotions, and aligning one's lifestyle with these seasonal rhythms is integral to holistic well-being.

Spring, the season of renewal and growth, corresponds with the Wood element in TCM. During this period, the liver and gallbladder are considered primary organ systems, and activities that support their function are encouraged. Spring rituals often involve detoxifying herbs and foods, such as dandelion greens and green tea, into one's diet. Movement practices like Tai Chi or Yoga can aid in promoting the smooth flow of Qi, ensuring a harmonious transition from the dormant winter to the vibrancy of spring.

As spring transitions to summer, the element of Fire takes center stage, aligning with the heart and small intestine organ systems. Summer rituals focus on balancing the heart's energy and embracing the season's warmth. Light, cooling foods like watermelon and cucumber become staples, and outdoor activities that harness the expansive power of summer, such as walking or swimming, are encouraged. Emotionally, summer is associated with joy, and practices that uplift the spirit, like spending time in nature, become essential.

Autumn marks the shift to the metal element associated with the lungs and large intestines. During harvest and reflection, autumn rituals involve nourishing the lungs with pears and apples and adopting practices that support introspection, such as journaling or meditation. Letting go of what is no longer needed, both physically and emotionally, aligns with the essence of autumn. It is a time to release, creating space for new energies to enter.

The transition to winter, associated with the Water element, invites inward turning and energy conservation. Winter rituals prioritize nourishing the kidneys, the primary organ system of the season, with warming, nutrient-dense foods like soups and stews. Practices emphasizing rest and rejuvenation, such as adequate sleep and gentle exercises like Qi Gong, support the body's ability to preserve vital energy during the colder months.

In addition to these seasonal rituals, TCM places significant emphasis on Qigong, an ancient Chinese exercise that combines movement, breath, and meditation. Qigong, often translated as "energy work," involves gentle, flowing movements that mimic the patterns of nature. Qigong practitioners work to balance and develop their Qi, which helps them develop a strong connection with the natural forces in their environment. Qigong is a spiritual practice that expands on the idea that one's internal energies and the exterior forces of nature are interconnected. It is not merely a physical workout.

Feng Shui, another essential component of TCM, extends the connection with nature to the living environment. Translated as "wind-water," Feng Shui is an ancient art that harmonizes energy flow in one's surroundings. By aligning the placement of objects, colors, and elements within a space with the principles of Feng Shui, individuals seek to create an environment that supports balance and positive energy. This practice enhances the aesthetic quality of living spaces and contributes to a sense of harmony and well-being.

TCM also advocates for people to spend time in parks, on hikes, or in gardens to fully immerse themselves in nature. The body's Qi balance is influenced by regular exposure to natural elements, which are potent sources of healing energy found in nature.

In the framework of TCM, establishing a connection with nature and the seasons is a dynamic and adaptive practice rather than static or inflexible. It entails becoming aware of the minute fluctuations in energy that occur both within and externally and making decisions consciously that follow the natural world's cyclical patterns. This interdependence encourages us to recognize the knowledge that the seasons hold and is a constant reminder that, like nature, our bodies and minds are constantly changing. Using these customs and routines, people set out on a path toward a holistic way of life, aligning with the cycles of the seasons and developing a strong bond with the vital forces of the planet.

Exploring the Spiritual Essence of Herbal Medicine

Exploring the spiritual essence of herbal medicine unveils a dimension that transcends the physical attributes of plants and delves into the profound interplay between nature, healing, and the human spirit. Rooted in ancient traditions and holistic philosophies, this exploration reveals herbal medicine as a collection of remedies and a conduit for connecting with the spiritual energies inherent in the plant kingdom.

In traditional herbalism, the spiritual essence of plants is often intertwined with cultural and indigenous beliefs, forming a sacred connection between humans and the natural world. Various cultures around the globe, from Native American traditions to Ayurvedic practices, have revered herbs for their physical healing properties and the spiritual wisdom they are believed to impart. This spiritual aspect emphasizes that plants possess a living energy, or spirit, that can facilitate profound emotional, mental, and spiritual healing.

Herbalists often approach the gathering and preparation of medicinal herbs with a reverence that goes beyond the mechanical process. Harvesting plants is seen as a sacred exchange, where practitioners express gratitude for the plant's offerings and seek permission before harvesting. This respectful relationship acknowledges the reciprocity between humans and the plant kingdom, fostering a spiritual connection that transcends the transactional nature of herbalism.

Herbal medicine in spiritual practices is prevalent in many ancient cultures. Shamans and healers often employ specific herbs as allies in rituals, ceremonies, and energetic healing. The smoke from burning herbs, known as smudging, is a widely recognized spiritual practice in indigenous cultures aimed at purifying the energy of spaces, individuals, or ceremonial tools. Herbs like sage, cedar, and sweetgrass are chosen for their physical cleansing properties and their perceived ability to dispel negative energies and invite positive spiritual influences.

In Western herbal traditions, certain herbs are considered not only for their physical benefits but also for their vibrational qualities. Flower essences, for example, capture the energetic imprint of flowers in water through solarization or boiling. These essences are believed to hold the plant's spiritual and emotional healing properties, resonating with specific aspects of the human psyche. Practitioners often incorporate flower essences into spiritual practices, meditation, or energy healing sessions to address underlying emotional or spiritual imbalances.

In the framework of Ayurveda and traditional Chinese medicine (TCM), herbalism also acknowledges the spiritual aspect of healing. Herbs are chosen in TCM based on their physiological effects and compatibility with particular organs, meridians, and spiritual attributes. Herbal treatments address these deeper facets of well-being since Traditional Chinese Medicine (TCM) takes a holistic approach, acknowledging that emotional or spiritual imbalances can also present as physical illnesses.

Herbs are seen by the ancient Indian medical system Ayurveda as carriers of prana, or life force. According to Ayurveda, an herb's flavor, energetics, and doshas (biological energies) all have a spiritual component. Herbal remedies restore equilibrium to the body, mind, and spirit by balancing the doshas. Herbs are prized for their capacity to deepen the spiritual bond, induce a sense of serenity and centeredness, and heal physically, including holy basil and ashwagandha.

Beyond specific cultural or traditional practices, exploring the spiritual essence of herbal medicine invites individuals to develop a personal relationship with plants. This may involve practices such as plant meditation, where individuals connect with the energy of a particular herb through focused contemplation. Engaging with plants in this way can deepen intuition, a heightened awareness of one's surroundings, and an expanded sense of spiritual connection.

Herbal medicine is also intertwined with the concept of plant spirit medicine, an approach that recognizes the consciousness and wisdom inherent in plants. Practitioners of plant spirit medicine engage in deep communion with plants, seeking guidance, healing, and insight directly from the plant's spirit. This approach involves developing a spiritual relationship with specific plants or trees, allowing their wisdom to guide and support personal and collective healing journeys.

In conclusion, exploring the spiritual essence of herbal medicine unveils a profound dimension of healing that extends beyond the physical properties of plants. It invites individuals to view herbs not just as remedies but as allies in the journey of personal and spiritual growth. Whether rooted in indigenous traditions, Western herbalism, or ancient healing systems, the spiritual connection with herbs fosters a sense of reverence, gratitude, and interconnectedness with the natural world. Developing a deeper awareness of the complex dance between spirituality, nature, and the human experience, as well as tapping into the healing energies of plants, can be accomplished by embracing the spiritual essence of herbal medicine.

CONCLUSION

In the final pages of "Roots of Wellness: Exploring Chinese Herbal Medicine - Traditional Wisdom for Modern Living," readers are immersed in a unique blend of ancient wisdom and modern perspectives. This e-book stands out as an in-depth guide and a profound exploration of traditional healing practices, effectively bridging the gap between time-honored wisdom and the needs of contemporary living.

The e-book begins by carefully dissecting the fundamentals of Chinese herbal medicine, covering the concepts of Yin and Yang, the Five Elements, and the crucial idea of Qi. It establishes a robust framework, enabling readers to appreciate the interconnectedness of the body, mind, and environment—an essential understanding for anyone seeking a holistic approach to wellness.

The heart of the e-book lies in its comprehensive examination of various Chinese herbs and their therapeutic properties. From ginseng and astragalus to goji berries and chrysanthemum, each herb is presented as a thread in the intricate tapestry of Chinese herbal medicine. Readers are guided through the nuances of herbal formulations, learning how combinations can be tailored to address specific imbalances and promote overall well-being.

More than just a compendium of herbs, the e-book unfolds as a practical guide to herbal formulation. It empowers readers to apply the wisdom of traditional Chinese medicine in their everyday lives. Easy-to-follow recipes and helpful tips encourage individuals to incorporate these ancient remedies into their modern routines, fostering a sense of self-care that aligns with the natural rhythms of life.

As the e-book progresses, it navigates the terrain of preventive healthcare, emphasizing the importance of balance and harmony in maintaining wellness. It underscores the role of Chinese herbal medicine in treating ailments and cultivating resilience and vitality. This paradigm shift resonates with the growing interest in proactive and holistic healthcare approaches.

The e-book draws upon the vast reservoir of traditional Chinese medical knowledge to address contemporary health challenges. It explores the potential of Chinese herbs in supporting the immune system, managing stress, and promoting longevity, offering practical insights that bridge the ancient with the urgent needs of the present.

The last chapter, "Roots of Wellness," emphasizes how Chinese herbal treatment is timeless and can be tailored to the intricacies of contemporary life. It encourages readers to adopt a perspective that values harmony, balance, and a close bond with the natural world. This ethos transcends cultural boundaries and resonates with individuals seeking a more integrative and mindful approach to health.

In essence, "Roots of Wellness" is not merely a guidebook but an invitation to embark on a transformative journey toward holistic well-being. It invites readers to rediscover the roots of their health and vitality, drawing from the deep well of traditional Chinese medicine. As the final chapter unfolds, readers are equipped with knowledge and a newfound appreciation for the ancient wisdom that continues to offer profound insights into the art of living well in the modern age. The e-book stands as a beacon, guiding individuals towards a path of wellness rooted in tradition yet illuminated by the possibilities of the future.

Thank you for buying and reading/listening to our book. If you found this book useful/helpful please take a few minutes and leave a review on the platform where you purchased our book. Your feedback matters greatly to us.

www.ingramcontent.com/pod-product-compliance
Lightning Source LLC
LaVergne TN
LVHW012025060526
838201LV00061B/4456